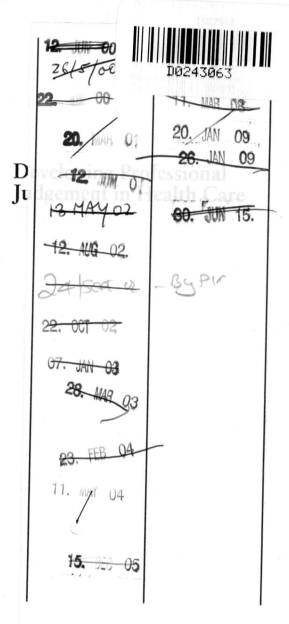

D0243063

12. JUN 00
26/5/00
22. JUN 00
20. MAR 01
12. JUN 01
18 MAY 02
12. AUG 02
24 SEP 02 — By Pir
22. OCT 02
07. JAN 03
28. MAR 03
23. FEB 04
11. MAY 04
15. DEC 05

11. MAR 08
20. JAN 09
26. JAN 09
30. JUN 15.

WHJ 1207

Books should be returned to the SDH Library on or before
the date stamped above unless a renewal has been arranged.

Salisbury District Hospital Library

Telephone: Salisbury (01722) 336262   extn. 4432 / 33
Out of hours answer machine in operation

D
Ju
Developing Professional
Judgement in Health Care

Developing Professional Judgement in Health Care

Learning Through the Critical Appreciation of Practice

Edited by

Della Fish PhD, MA, MEd, BA Hons, Dip Ed

Consultant in Educational and Professional Development
Honorary Research Fellow, School of Education,
Exeter University

Colin Coles PhD, MA, BSc Hons

Professor of Medical Education,
Institute of Health and Community Studies,
Bournemouth University

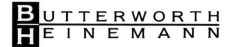
BUTTERWORTH
HEINEMANN

Butterworth-Heinemann
Linacre House, Jordan Hill, Oxford OX2 8DP
225 Wildwood Avenue, Woburn, MA 01801–2041
A division of Reed Educational and Professional Publishing Ltd

℞ A member of the Reed Elsevier plc group

OXFORD   BOSTON   JOHANNESBURG
MELBOURNE   NEW DELHI   SINGAPORE

First published 1998

© Reed Educational and Professional Publishing Ltd 1998

All rights reserved. No part of this publication may be reproduced in
any material form (including photocopying or storing in any medium
by electronic means and whether or not transiently or incidentally to
some other use of this publication) without the written permission of
the copyright holder except in accordance with the provisions of the
Copyright, Designs and Patents Act 1988 or under the terms of a
licence issued by the Copyright Licensing Agency Ltd, 90 Tottenham
Court Road, London, England W1P 9HE. Applications for the
copyright holder's written permission to reproduce any part of this
publication should be addressed to the publishers.

British Library Cataloguing in Publication Data

Developing professional judgement in health care:learning
    through the critical appreciation of practice
    1.   Clinical medicine 2.   Medical care
    I   Fish, Della II   Coles, Colin
    616

ISBN 0 7506 3123 6

Library of Congress Cataloguing in Publication Data

Developing professional judgement in health care:learning through
    the critical appreciation of practice/edited by Della Fish, Colin
    Coles.
        p.   cm.
    Includes bibliographical references and index.
    ISBN 0 7506 3123 6
    1   Medicine – Decision making.   I   Fish, Della.   II   Coles, Colin
    [DNLM: 1   Professional Practice.   2   Medicine.   3   Judgement.   W
87 D489]
    R723.5.D48
    610 – dc21   97–30471
                                                                    CIP

Printed and bound in Great Britain by
Biddles Ltd, Guildford and Kings Lynn

Contents

Contributors

Clive Andrewes
Clive works in the Institute of Health and Community Studies at
Bournemouth University in the position of Co-ordinator of Practice
Development. This post involves developing collaborative projects
between academic staff and clinical staff in health and social care
settings. Prior to this he was involved with education as a course
leader to undergraduate programmes in nursing in Leeds and
London. He has published books on medical nursing and contributes chapters on, amongst other things, children and dying and
gastroenterology.

Judith Chapman
Judith, who is both a British subject and a Canadian citizen, is a
lecturer in physiotherapy at Southampton University. She trained at
King's College Hospital, London and worked there for two years
before going to Canada. There, she worked in hospitals and then
joined the staff at McMaster Health Science Centre, specialising in
rheumatology. She later became a clinical instructor, placing and
supervising students, and after completing a masters degree in
health sciences, she became a member of faculty in the McMaster
degree programme and a research therapist in rheumatology. Her
interests are in problem based learning and the assessment of
learning.

Colin Coles
Colin's academic base is the Institute of Health and Community
Studies at Bournemouth University, where he holds a personal chair

in medical education. From here he undertakes commissioned workshops and research projects across a wide range of health professional and multi-professional groups in the UK and overseas, particularly in the field of educating educators. His academic background was originally in psychology and biological sciences, and he has taught in schools, colleges of education and universities. In 1994 he co-edited *Learning in Medicine,* Scandinavian Universities Press (Oxford University Press), and contributes widely to academic journals, books and professional publications. He is a member of the Standing Committee for Postgraduate Medical and Dental Education and the British Medical Association's Board of Medical Education.

Della Fish

Della was Principal Lecturer in Education at what is now Brunel University, and is an Honorary Research Fellow in Education at Exeter University. She works as a consultant on educational and professional development, offering workshops across the caring professions. She holds a masters and a doctoral degree in English and a masters degree in education and has taught in schools and in higher education. Deep interest in course design led her into her consultancy work. She has been an external examiner for undergraduate courses in education, occupational therapy and physiotherapy and for masters degrees in education. She has published books on education for the professions, and carried out contract research for and sat on steering committees of major national projects in nursing.

Crissi Gallagher

Crissi trained in occupational therapy at Oxford and gained a masters degree in education at Southampton University in 1992. She is a lecturer at the School of Occupational Therapy and Physiotherapy at Southampton University. Prior to this she had experience of training and development within the National Health Service, and worked clinically in a variety of mental health specialties, including In- and Day Patient Rehabilitation.

Richard Hillier

Richard has been a consultant in palliative care in the National Health Service since 1976. He has played a key role in the development of palliative care by health care workers in hospitals and in the community. He has also been involved in developing specialist palliative care teaching and research in the UK and abroad. His recent initiation into reflective practice has helped him to examine long-standing issues and difficulties in his own work with a new enthusiasm and initiative, which has revitalised both his practice and his teaching.

Sheila Reading

Sheila is a lecturer in the School of Nursing and Midwifery at Southampton University. She has developed and now teaches a research skills module for registered nurses, midwives and health visitors carrying out undergraduate studies. Her main interests are in developing research teaching strategies for the optimal benefit of practitioners, clinical practice and client/nursing care, and encouraging dialogue about the role of a research dissertation for professional practitioners.

Rosemary Richardson

Rosemary is a lecturer in the School of Nursing and Midwifery at the University of Southampton. Her teaching commitments include community related aspects of pre- and post-registration nurse education courses at certificate, diploma and degree level. She has a masters degree in education and is currently a doctoral student. She is particularly interested in increasing the understanding and development of practice through reflective and critically analytical approaches.

Glossary

CQI	continuous quality improvement
DoH	Department of Health
DOTP	Director of Occupational Therapy Practice
ENB	English National Board of Nursing, Midwifery and Health Visiting
GP	general practitioner
HMSO	Her Majesty's Stationery Office
IPR	individual performance review
MRC	Medical Research Council
NFER	National Foundation for Educational Research
NHS	National Health Service
NVQ	National Vocational Qualification
PA	professional artistry
TQM	total quality management
TR	technical rational
UKCC	United Kingdom Central Council for Nursing, Midwifery and Health Visiting

Acknowledgements

We are particularly grateful to Rosemary Barnitt, Senior Lecturer in Occupational Therapy at Southampton University, for permission to hold two major workshops at the University's School of Occupational Therapy and Physiotherapy, and for hospitality provided, and to Richard Hillier, Medical Director of Countess Mountbatten House, for providing shelter and sustenance for all other meetings.

We acknowledge with gratitude the help and support during the preparation of this publication from Susan Devlin, senior medical editor for Butterworth–Heinemann, who brought a human touch to her role in liaising with us, provided hospitality, and came to meet all the writers.

This book would not have reached the publisher without the dedication of Jean Douglas and Evelyn Usher who, with endless patience and good humour, meticulously corrected drafts and proof-read.

Any opinions expressed are entirely those of the authors and are in no way associated with any institution or official body for which any of us works.

Della Fish and Colin Coles

Part One

Towards a Re-vision of Professional Practice

Della Fish and Colin Coles

Chapter 1

Professionalism eroded: professionals under siege

Our starting points: a view of professionalism

Professionals are under siege. Everywhere in the developed world they are being challenged. They feel threatened and defensive, overloaded and highly pressurised. This is as true in health care as in other professions. They feel let down by the public they serve, their professional bodies to whom they hold allegiance, and by the politicians who provide the fiscal and policy frameworks within which they practise. As we write this book at the end of the twentieth century, arguably as never before professionals feel a need to stand up and be counted.

We set out to write this book with a very strong sense of purpose. Working over the years in education and in health care, we have become acutely aware of the concerns which professional people voice. And for anything we have felt able to achieve with these professionals at the time, by holding seminars, running staff development workshops, conducting research projects, writing reports, sitting on national and local committees, we frequently felt frustrated at not being able to go further. We knew that there was more to do, we sensed we should be able to do more to help them to face their everyday challenges. Yet we felt unable to achieve very much in the few hours (or even few days) we could spend on one project or another. We knew there was (and is) something quite fundamental that needs to be addressed, something to do with professional education and development, with how professionals are helped to become professionals and to maintain their professionalism, that has rarely been dealt with satisfactorily up to now. How could we help our colleagues (and perhaps ourselves) to cope with the present times, and move forward to the future with greater confidence?

Until very recently, professionals felt that they held a position of considerable trust. Society gave them freedom and autonomy within which professionals were allowed to do what they considered right, at the right time, in the right way. Professionals are indeed allowed to undertake certain procedures, to act in certain ways, and to discuss certain matters with members of the public which, if carried out by anyone else, would at least cause affront and at worst be indictable offences. All societies entrust these functions to certain of its members. Professionals are expected to be trustworthy, and in their turn they expect to receive the public's trust in them.

In return professionals were prepared to undertake a lengthy period of education, which for many was particularly protracted in order for them to gain higher professional qualifications. They were prepared to commit considerable amounts of time and effort to their work. They did not clock watch, or do it for the money. They did more than was asked of them. They went further than their contracts of employment. All because they felt it was right to do so. They were professionals. They stood somewhat apart from the rest of society. They took on a professional role. And in recompense for their personal commitment, society gave them professional status, a greater than average income. For this society expected high ethical standards of course, and the maintenance of confidentiality. The tacit agreement was this: society would trust professionals if they could be trusted.

Society also recognised (perhaps more in the past than at the present time) that professional practice is difficult to define. Professionals must do what they think fit. Society would not ask any questions. It saw that what a professional actually does cannot always be planned. The 'right thing to do' emerges in the course of the professional's contact with patients or clients. Indeed, those professional actions that require the highest level of expertise are those that simply cannot be predicted in advance. Professionals are educated, held in high esteem, and well paid, largely so that they are able to make appropriate judgements in situations where there is no right answer, where difficult choices must be made, where there is a moral dimension to the practitioner's actions.

This symbiotic relationship between professionals and public is of course based on an 'understanding'. It has never (until now) been formally codified into a contract. It was unstated, as we have said, a tacit agreement. And this understanding was an assumed one. When a member of the public approached a professional for help or advice, the assumptions they both made about their relationship pre-empted that contract. There was no need for the professional to state his or her credentials (though they might display certificates indicating their qualifications), and members of the public knew (or thought they knew) what a particular professional could do for them, and they trusted (to a greater or lesser extent) the professional's ability to practise effectively and efficiently in their interests.

Of course there are, and always have been, abuses to this trust. Some professionals have been guilty of wrong-doing. Some have neglected the public's wishes, or not met their needs. Some have failed to keep up to date, have taken their qualifications to be a 'ticket for life'. Some failed to base their practice on the best possible evidence. Some practised idiosyncratically and in an unsubstantiated manner. Some misused the power of their position – "do as the nurse says" or "you must obey doctor's orders". And some have used the powers given to them by society to protect their own and their profession's interests. Malpractice has been 'covered up' by professionals 'sticking together' and by 'closing ranks'.

Then there is the problem of litigation or at least the increased threat of it. Throughout the developed world professional people are fearful of the legal consequences of their mistakes. Where it used to be recognised that these might occur because the work was highly complex, now the public senses that they can be compensated, obtain some recompense, make something out of it. This has the effect of making professional practice more tentative, more conservative. Medical people, for example, will investigate a condition more, carry out further tests, and rely less on their judgement – to be on the safe side but also to cover themselves.

Yet at the present time the authority professionals once had – their inborn sense of doing the right things, at the right time, in the right way – is being challenged. Public trust is no longer there – or so it seems – and governments of all political shades (and in most developed countries) increasingly want value for money, more for less. Politicians, who in their turn desire the public's trust in them, sense the public wants something more (or different) from professional people.

So why do we say that professionals are under siege? What is causing this? Why has the public's trust become eroded? And why now?

Examining the siege further

One answer is that professionals in the past were indeed given a blank cheque, carte blanche, to practise as they wished. But in a society where there is increasing competitiveness, rising living standards, where people have much greater disposable incomes than ever before, there is perhaps a sense of resentment that professionals should be given so much autonomy without a correspondingly high level of accountability to accompany it. The blanket trust, the almost blind faith that people once had in professionals, is no longer socially acceptable.

Another reason for the siege is that a more educated and technologically sophisticated public no longer believes that professional work is so different from theirs, of such a higher order of magnitude compared with the actions they carry out themselves. And a wealthier public, a consumer society, is more prepared to ask questions of professionals and to demand answers. Greater wealth means more power, and people spend more of their money privately on homes, schools, transport, and health. There is more choice, a greater range of options, people can get what they want. And the public applies the same thinking to professionals, who increasingly in their eyes are now seen to be no different from themselves – people holding down a job, living ordinary lives – which in many ways is absolutely true. The mystique surrounding the professional has all but disappeared.

In health care – as elsewhere – costs are rising. Technological advances, and the increasing range of treatment options available, together with the costs of actually providing the care itself, are spiralling upwards across the world (in developed and developing countries alike). And governments must pay the bills. They are held accountable by the public to meet their demands. Yet health care is racing away with resources. Some political check must be placed on this inexorable rise. Or at least some plausible explanation must be given to the public as to why people cannot have what they demand or what they see others getting.

In areas of technological advance health professionals feel challenged too regarding ethical issues. In vitro fertilisation, selective termination of pregnancy, and euthanasia are all issues in which the public now feels it has a voice, that these are areas that should not be left to professionals alone to resolve. Professional authority is being questioned, and professional power challenged.

There is too a blurring of the traditional distinctions between the professions. The work once carried out only by doctors is now performed by others. (Sometimes this causes public concern, as in press reports of nurses performing surgical operations.) But there is universally a downgrading of professional tasks, and some professionals wonder how it will end, what the cost to human suffering will be, or where this will ultimately leave professional identity.

The political response to these societal changes has been to demand greater accountability of the professions. Health care is now contracted, and these contracts go way beyond the tacit understanding between professionals and their public we spoke of earlier. Contracted care says in effect: you professionals are asked to undertake certain activities, in a certain time, to a certain standard, for which you will be paid a certain amount. Contracts focus on what is measurable – the outcomes of care – and they favour acute rather than chronic illness. They are difficult to construct in chronic and long term illness, and in contracting for the professional–client relationship. But more than this, it is the politicians who have set out the policy frameworks for care. Guidelines and protocols have been developed in an attempt to ensure that health care practice is performed to the highest standards, to keep professionals up to date, and frequently these have been devised by people who are not health professionals themselves, often by bureaucrats.

Of course, these contracts inevitably restrict the professional's autonomy. They seriously question the professional's right to conduct his or her practice as he or she sees fit. They deeply challenge professionals' personal commitment to maintaining their own standards. And above all they threaten professionals' long held (and strenuously coveted) belief in self-regulation. Quite understandably a professional might say "I've received an extensive education to get where I am, why do you now face me with all these controls and restrictions on my professional actions? Don't you trust me any more?" And the answer (implied of course, not made explicit from society) is an emphatic "No!" So it is no wonder that some professionals have called for a return to a world where they were told 'here is £x million – do what you can with it' (Hopkins and Solomon, 1996, p. 477).

Perhaps the greatest problem though for professionals is that they are an easy target. Much professional work (including decision-making like diagnostic reasoning, clinical reasoning and professional judgement) is carried out intuitively – one might even say unconsciously. Professionals feel they are doing the right thing in the right circumstances but are often not fully aware of what they are doing and more particularly why they are doing it. We are not saying that professionals do not know what they are doing. Nor are we saying they are ignorant of their practice. How could we? We would claim to be professionals ourselves. What we are saying is this – and it is central to our argument in this book and underpins our reasons for embarking upon this project. If stopped in the middle of some action or procedure, professionals would be hard pressed to explain their knowledge base for practising in a particular way or how they acquired the expertise to do so. They would not know what it meant to be the professional they undoubtedly are. They would have difficulty in saying what was the nature of their expertise.

Our claim for saying, then, that professionals are under siege is this: at a time when they are being challenged to account *for* their actions and the judgements that lie at the base of them, professionals seem grossly unprepared to give an account *of* them. Much professional practice 'comes with experience', and it is almost impossible to pass that experience on to others. Yet to describe one's professional judgements as being 'a hunch' or 'a gut feeling' demeans those actions, and for professionals to use these terms as justification for their actions is as unsatisfactory to them as it is to others. They entirely fail to convey to the public the deep and complex nature of professional practice, nor do they anywhere nearly justify the need for a lengthy and expensive education or a high salary. And these are weak terms which cut little ice with politicians. Is 'intuition' the only justification a professional can give in return for an unquestioning trust? Clearly not! Yet professionals have few other ways of explaining the nature of their professionalism. They do not know what it is, where it comes from, or how they acquired it.

All of this seems to suggest that the siege which professionals experience is the consequence of outside factors. Real though these undoubtedly are, professionals are also under siege from within themselves. Being separate from the rest of society gives professionals autonomy but it also brings considerable isolation. Making professional decisions of a high order may carry with it greater social respect and higher remuneration than others receive for more mundane work but it means too that 'the buck stops with them'. Who can they turn to for support, except other professionals who are themselves facing their own personal challenges? Even leaders of a professional team are isolated in their leadership role. And some professionals' practice is isolated in even a literal sense – they work alone – in consulting rooms for example.

But many professionals today also feel besieged because they sense their profession is no longer a vocation. They had been attracted to this work because of its intrinsic worth, because of the service they felt they were able to provide to society, because of the good they could do. Yet they now see their colleagues (and particularly their trainees) eschewing these very principles that gave meaning and substance to work which demanded long hours and a sense of personal commitment. These days professional work is more of a job than a vocation. And if that element of their pro-fessionalism is eroded, what is left? If their junior colleagues are no longer prepared to put their work before their family or social life (as they did) what can the future possibly hold? If they can no longer defend their professionalism to others (or even to themselves) in terms of 'vocation', what does it mean to be a professional?

The problem, we believe, is not that professionals are any different from (or any worse than) they ever were. Far from it. Professionals are even more expert, even more highly tuned, even more highly pressed and pressurised to do the right thing. It is not that professionals work any less, or work less well. The reverse is the case. No, the problem is that professionals cannot say what is the basis of their professionalism. They do not have the where-withal to understand their practice. They never have had. The problem is not new. Professionals have probably always faced these tensions because of their very special relationship with society.

Quite probably too these tensions come and go. At certain times they are greater than at others. And at the present time, reflecting other more general movements in society, these pressures are greater than ever.

Our intentions for the book

Our claim is then that most professionals (in the way they have been or are being educated) have not been helped to understand the nature of their professional practice, and they are not encouraged, not given the time or opportunity, to do so in their present work. So we have written this book because we believe there is a way forward in responding to professionals' deep-seated need to understand (and account for) their professionalism. What is more, we believe that the understanding which professionals can thus gain is sounder and more convincing than basing one's professional practice on a sense of vocation. We are convinced (by our experience before writing this book and even more so in its preparation) that there is a very real basis to professional expertise that professionals can (and should) get nearer to the bottom of, and we believe that the work we describe in this book is a way of achieving that understanding. We say 'nearer to understanding' here because, for reasons we outline in Chapter 3, we subscribe to the view that there will always be some mystery at the very heart of a professional's work.

And we have written this book for another, we believe crucial, reason. There is a view, firmly held in some quarters, that the way forward for professions, the direction needed for development, is through the discovery of new knowledge. The belief is that progress occurs when we know new things. And the principle means for achieving this is research. So professional people have engaged in research to discover things they did not know before. That is not wrong, of course. New knowledge is vital for expanding professional activity. Our concern, however, is this: very little research has been carried out into professional practice, into what the basis is for the actions professionals take. Our interest in writing this book is to explore ways of undertaking research which enable professional people (like ourselves) to understand our practice and by this means to refine and improve it.

How the book is arranged

In the second part of this book we present a set of case studies each of which is focused upon a piece of personal professional practice and the specific actions and judgements involved in it. These are drawn from a wide range of health care professions and offer readers examples of how professionals, with whom we worked over a one year period, have used certain ideas and means (which we discussed together as they proceeded) to unlock their practice, and how as a result they have grown to understand it and themselves better. This is the very heart of the book and drives its major purposes.

This work – that of our contributors and our own – has involved an investment of time and disciplined enquiry which makes what we want to call the critical appreciation of professional practice as rigorous, scholarly and professional as any form of scientific re-search, and more especially of greater relevance to professional development. We argue that this approach of looking closely at the stories we encouraged people to tell and investigating *them* (rather than rushing away from them to create or capture new data, as happens in other research) is more likely than is empirical enquiry to lead to an understanding of professional practice. While scien-tific research is important in creating new knowledge in health care, practice research and development are vital too.

But we on our part go further. We have not, like outside research-ers, simply conducted case study research into people's practice. We do not see practice development research in that way. Rather we have engaged a group of health professionals in the critical appreciation of *their own* practice, and we hope to demonstrate in this book that this approach, which some call insider practitioner research (see Reed and Procter, 1995), is a key to a major form of professional self-development, and is more valuable in every way than any training imposed from outside, or any scientific research, in developing professionals' practice. And we do so because we believe that, whatever contribution scientific research might make to the treatment of disease, professional self-development is central to the improvement of health care itself.

In this book then we will consider carefully what is meant by common enough terms such as critical appreciation, reflection, deliberation, case study, various kinds of research, and even professional education. This we attempt in Part One of the book.

Chapter 2 looks at the practical basis, and Chapter 3 the theoretical basis of our practice. Chapter 4 then describes the approach we adopted with our contributors and the thinking that lies beneath it.

Part Two of the book offers the reflective and deliberative case studies themselves. Each individual professional's path through his or her enquiry is different. Yet there are principles and processes in common across these cases and which, importantly, are common across a wide range of professions too. In Part Three we respond to these through a process of critical appreciation which at the same time illustrates how such an approach can extend the understandings which emerge from reflection and deliberation. Finally, in Part Four we consider various ways forward for practitioner education and practitioner research.

Readership

We are writing for a wide audience of health care professionals. It is not a book in which we expect the reader to learn about and be caught up with the *detail* of other professionals' concerns. Rather, we intend the reader to use this book as a means of thinking about his or her *own* practice, and as a help in considering through what processes he or she might better understand it. Whether these particular cases relate directly to the reader's profession or not, therefore, we trust they will be of value in terms of what they say about the *development* of a health care professional. We hope that they will motivate the reader to focus upon and develop his or her own practice (and perhaps the exercise of professional judgement within it) and to explore the potential for so doing of the processes of reflection, deliberation and appreciation.

We are writing this book with three broad groups of readers in mind. First, there are students of health care. As we shall argue in the next chapter, professional education leaves much to be desired. Students are often overloaded with content, much of it dealing with the scientific basis of disease management rather than health care practice. Many students find difficulty in understanding the relevance of much of the theory they have to learn, and find difficulty too in applying it in a practical setting. Their world seems more about passing academic examinations than learning how to practise. Many undergraduates courses too, these days, contain projects where students must undertake some kind of research into health care. Yet the scientific model of research (often held up to students as the only legitimate approach) does not ring true to them in the world of practice they are beginning to experience. We hope to show students an alternative way of researching their practice.

Next we are writing for health care practitioners themselves. Like students, the newly qualified find difficulty in applying their theoretical knowledge and in adjusting to the working world of full time practice. And as if this were not enough, at the same time they must continue studying for specialist qualifications. They also begin to recognise that practice is much more messy than they were led to believe, and worse, they see this as their own fault – they cannot have studied sufficiently well during their initial training. We aspire to show them this is not true. The fault, if there is one, lies in the lack of support they receive in understanding and coping with the inevitably messy world of practice.

As fully qualified specialist practitioners they need to keep up to date and to incorporate new findings and approaches into their practice. Now, the burden of blame shifts from themselves to the system – if they cannot find answers to the problems of practice themselves, what are the managers or politicians doing about it? So we are writing too for expert practitioners, to help them understand their practice and to cope with the demands of accountability we spoke of earlier.

The final group for whom we are writing comprises health care teachers. Some are full time academics, perhaps with clinical responsibilities. Some are practitioners with teaching responsibilities. Very few are qualified educationalists. Yet they recognise the problems facing their students and trainees. They see motivation slip away, and commitment to care seriously challenged by the day-to-day realities of professional practice for which professional education is only an imperfect preparation and support. But as teachers they have few answers. Governmental and professional pressures to reform curricula and training programmes are of little help (but are merely an added burden) and teachers are suspicious that the motives of educational reformers are not entirely in their students' or their profession's interests. On top of this they, like their students, must undertake research to survive in a world that more and more values facts and outcomes than resolving conjectures and dilemmas or understanding professional practice.

References

Hopkins, A. and Solomon, K. (1996). Can contracts drive clinical care? *British Medical Journal*, **313**, 447–448.

Reed, J. and Procter, S. (eds.) (1995). *Practitioner Research in Health Care: the Inside Story*. Chapman and Hall.

Chapter 2

Uncertainty in a certain world: professionals in health care

Introduction

In Chapter 1 we described today's challenges to professional practice, and to practitioners themselves. We saw how the public trust in professions has been eroded, partly through societal changes and partly through political pressures. There are increasing demands on professionals for accountability yet professional people feel unable to say what the precise basis is for those acts of professional practice that give professionalism its uniqueness – their professional judgements. We noted the failure of education to provide professionals with the wherewithal to justify their actions, and the equal failure of their current circumstances to provide resources for them to understand (and through that understanding to develop) their current practice.

In that opening chapter, then, we tried to depict a world our readers would recognise (that is, a world in which practitioners from all kinds of professions have to work). We showed it to be a troubled one, particularly at the present time. In this next chapter our focus shifts. As we pointed out earlier, what we have written here is the result of discussions we undertook with a group of professionals drawn from a range of health care professions whose contribution forms the heart of the book. Our task now is to explore (and to some extent explain) the context in which those colleagues have written their chapters. We felt is was important to look at the background of our colleagues and where they were coming from when they started out on this project, and we will do this by examining three key areas of their professional lives – their practice of health care, their past and present professional education, and the research tradition within which they work.

The practice of health care

The world of health care within which our colleagues work is changing rapidly. Spiralling costs, apparently insatiable public demand and technological advance all contribute to significant shifts in the nature of health care practice.

Many of the changes are no doubt in patients' best interests. There is a far greater focusing than ever before on people's actual needs, and not just those that the health professionals believe them to be. Patients' needs now take account of the views of relatives and non-professional carers too, and a much wider range of health professionals than before.

There is, as well, a greater community orientation of health care. No longer is the acute hospital the centre of health care activity. There is a greater recognition of the need to devote more resources to the needs of the chronically ill, and that chronic illness occurs in people's daily lives, where they live, and not just in hospitals. It affects how they live, whether (and how much) they can work, how mobile they are, how dependent they may be on others (including other health carers as well as social and public services).

There is recognition too that patients and carers have an enormous responsibility for their own health, and for the management of their condition when they are far beyond the reaches of health professionals. Whether or not a patient's condition is controlled or contained is more likely to rest with the patient or carer than with the health professional (Kaplan, Greenfield and Ware, 1989). While health professionals can diagnose conditions and provide a certain level of care, ultimately many patients and those closest to them must manage their condition for themselves.

These shifts (from acute to chronic care, from hospitals to community, from health professional centred to patient centred clinical management) have changed our colleagues' sense of professionalism enormously. No longer can they remain isolated. Co-operation and team working is essential. Multi-professional working – the breaking down of traditional professional boundaries – is demanded more and more. A key task for senior professionals today is that of co-ordinating and managing the care that the patient is receiving, irrespective of its location, of particular professional labels, or of traditional professional roles.

Another way in which our colleagues' world of health care has been changing (like that for other professionals too) concerns employment legislation. Greater attention is now given by both employers and employees to working conditions. Many of their workplaces are 'Investors in People', a national initiative which aims to develop the working environment and to provide support (and development) for the people who work within it. Discrimination on the grounds of race, gender or age is prohibited. Appointments procedures must be seen to be fair. Contracts of employment favour the employee more than the employer. Induction programmes for newly appointed staff are in place, and staff development programmes are on the increase. The working hours of professionals have improved, and the case of junior medical staff is a good example. Previously, doctors were expected to undertake any work necessary to complete the tasks in hand. This led to excessive working hours and even exploitation, and was only resolved with the involvement of their professional body (that is, the British Medical Association). One consequence is that health care is now seen more and more (not least by the professionals involved in it) as a job of work rather than a vocation. Contrary to our claims in the previous chapter, there is now more clock watching and more sense of contractual expectation and obligation than has previously been the case in health care.

But perhaps the greatest change, as we argued in the previous chapter, has been the introduction of contracts for purchasing and providing health. Probably this reflects a greater sense of consumerism in society at large but certainly it is an attempt by central government to control costs and increase efficiency. For the first time the actual costs of health care have been identified, and so too have the activities of the health professionals involved. But this has led to calls for more service to be provided for lower costs, for cost cutting, for efficiency savings.

Worse (as some health professionals see it), an emphasis on annual contracting for care means a focus on (and a need to respond to) short term demands, not longer term developments. Those areas of health care that are more difficult to define, such as social and psychological aspects of illness, continuing and palliative care, psychiatric and counselling support, are more difficult to defend. Activities favoured by the parties drawing up health care contracts are those that lead to clearly definable outcomes (and increasingly those that are measurable).

Some changes, reflecting the way resources are allocated, seemed to our colleagues to be drawn from a world of business and commerce, which they find alien to all they hold dear regarding professional practice. Contracting suggests certainty and predictability and an ability to state in a contract what will happen over a certain period of time. Professionals on the other hand know that in practice it is never that clear. Things will change, new priorities will emerge.

But perhaps the worst feature of contracting for our colleagues is the competitiveness it creates. If one group fails to get the contract, another will. So professionals must develop a 'competitive edge', be 'ahead of the game'. Co-operation and collaboration, key concepts they always held to be the basis of professional working, now seem outmoded and uncomfortable.

Perhaps the most significant concern for our colleagues is the way in which control of their professional practice is being exercised in the actual work they undertake. They recognise that they differ, one from another, in their approach and this is reinforced by their adopting different language. They also know that some activities they perform are more effective than others. Some are outdated and inefficient. Some are not based on available evidence. Some (or rather, many) have no guiding base at all (Greenhalgh, 1996). And in a health system of multi-professional working, where various professionals are each undertaking specific procedures, but each discussing them in the deliberately esoteric and closed language of their own individual professions, how can there be any certainty that what they actually do is appropriate, let alone safe? The answer has been for guidelines and protocols to be generated which set out how they are to conduct practical procedures. And our colleagues know that today the commissioners of health care are particularly interested in ensuring that the procedures they purchase meet the highest (and most efficient) standards.

So perhaps the greatest challenge has been to our colleagues' sense of professionalism – to the very basis of their professional practice – that as professionals they should conduct their practice as they see fit. And this challenge has been deeper than that and gone further in its implications. It has questioned the basis of their expertise. For them to say now that their practice and especially their judgement is the result of 'experience', or is 'intuitive', is no longer sufficient. It will no longer carry any weight.

So far in this chapter we have described the world of health care in which our colleagues are (or have been) practitioners. But they are health care practitioners in another world too – that of higher education. Each is involved in one way or another with teaching other health professionals. As well as being health care professionals they are also educators and academics, all of them holding university appointments. But the two universities from which our colleagues come are quite different, and it is important to highlight these differences in setting the context within which they make their contribution to this book.

One university has declared itself 'research led' and this fundamentally determines the perspective (and work patterns) of our colleagues based there. Research, as one would imagine, dominates their activities. Their focus is on research projects, grant applications and publications. Of course they must balance this with their teaching, but the emphasis of their work is clearly on research. Not least for them this dictates the criteria used for confirming appointments and in staff promotions.

The other university is newly established – a former polytechnic. Here teaching is (or has been until now) the dominant activity. Research is encouraged but teaching (and course development) is valued. So too is the development of clinical practice, which has a much greater emphasis here than in the university mentioned above. And these aspects of academic work form key elements in the appointment and promotions procedures (at least as much as and probably more than is found in many older universities).

Professional education

We turn now to our colleagues' experience of professional education to see how this too forms a context for their writing. In doing this we feel it is important to make two observations: they come from four different professions, and have a generation separating them. Yet from what they described to us as their educational experiences, the similarities far outweigh the differences. There are differences of course; medical education is perhaps the most academic and theoretical, emphasising the scientific (and particularly biological) basis of disease, and the focus is clearly on the diagnosis of illness. Nurse education is more focused on patient care, occupational therapy education emphasises social and psychological rehabilitation, and physiotherapy concentrates on the management of physical disability. There are also differences between the professional education our colleagues *experienced* and that which is offered today. It is therefore crucial to emphasise that we are describing their own experience in so far as it influences their current thinking (and working), and we are not discussing the present educational scene for the health professions.

What our colleagues most commonly experienced in their professional education was that it was modelled on the education of doctors. As we have said, there were differences reflecting the particular profession they were entering, but the model of medical education was the 'gold standard' to which the other professionals seemed to aspire. Doctors' education had by far the highest academic status, and was certainly the longest. And many of the teachers of the other professions were doctors or academics (or both).

A key feature of our colleagues' education was that it was intended as a preparation. Its purpose was to prepare them so they could practise in the health service. But as we shall see from their accounts (and in our discussion), this preparation left much to be desired. When they entered practice many felt grossly unprepared. And their subsequent specialist education, which was intended to provide them with further qualifications, did little for the development of their practice.

Most health care education comprises three distinct phases – undergraduate, postgraduate, and continuing education. While attempts have been made to make the educational programme 'seamless', largely these three remain separate. During the undergraduate phase as students they acquired a university degree in one field of health care or another. During the post-registration phase they learnt to work in health care, and they studied for higher specialist qualifications. Now, during their continuing education (covering by far the bulk of their careers), they attend courses, lectures and conferences, and they attempt to keep up with the journals, though (until very recently) little attention has been given to regulating (or even encouraging) their continuing development.

Our colleagues' undergraduate education was largely scientific. Generally, there was an emphasis on 'disease' rather than 'health' and certainly 'treatment' rather than 'care'. What was taught reflected 'discoveries' – that is, factual information and certainty. It was reductionist. It looked at finer and finer detail, at the parts rather than the whole.

Traditionally, health professional education separates theoretical and practical teaching, the former taking place in an academic (or scholastic) environment, the latter often in teaching hospitals focusing largely on acute conditions. Theory teachers are often university staff and practical teachers are health care practitioners.

Theory teaching for our colleagues was largely formal, with lectures the most common teaching method. Practical teaching on the other hand was mostly informal, at the bedside or in clinics, with a considerable amount of 'learning from experience'. With the exception of nursing, most of our colleagues' teachers were untrained for their teaching role. Both theoretical and practical teaching was 'authority based' – the teachers were both *an authority* in their subject and they were *in authority* over them as students.

So our colleagues were taught a lot of 'theory' (some more than others) because it was assumed they would need this knowledge in order to practise. And this theory was taught first – before they went into practice – because it was assumed you needed to have (what are often termed) 'the basics' before you could practise. Of course, this misunderstands (or misrepresents) the term 'basics' in several deep senses, which our colleagues only came to recognise later in their careers. Much of this 'theory' could never be applied to practice. A great deal of it they had forgotten anyway. And by being taught these so called 'basics' first, before they had much practical experience, they found great difficulty in seeing its relevance. They learnt (often by rote) these 'basics', and even passed examinations in them demonstrating how much they 'knew' (at that time). Yet paradoxically this 'knowing of the basics' was curiously unhelpful in preparing them for practice.

The educational assessments our colleagues experienced were largely for regulatory purposes and administered within clear legal frameworks. This is understandable in one sense – society demands protection from inadequate practitioners. In practice, however, these examinations became impersonal and formal. Indeed, our colleagues' experience of assessment was of hurdles to be surmounted, again with little relationship to practice and certainly not indicating their 'proficiency'.

Since qualifying, our colleagues have had a variety of educational experiences, some award bearing and providing further qualification. Several have completed masters courses in education. Much of their recent education has been less formal, often of shorter duration. Their in-service education, where it happened at all, has tended to be related to specific aspects of their practice. Some of this has involved other professional groups, but like much of the remainder of their education it has been uni-professional.

Before starting the project, all our colleagues knew, in varying degrees, about 'reflection on practice'. They were aware of the concept and current interest in it as an aspect of professional education. One had considerable experience of reflective teaching for undergraduates, and of reflective groups for practitioners in practice development. Yet some of the others were unsure what it meant in practice or what it involved. One or two were openly sceptical about its usefulness, particularly for themselves.

The research traditions

Research is a further element of our colleagues' experience that has strongly influenced their professional lives, and surfaces in the accounts of their practice they contribute to this book. Undeniably, in health care the most dominant research tradition is the scientific one, and some claim this to be the only true form of research. But there are others which are becoming increasingly common in health care. And since our colleagues are aware of the existence of these research approaches we feel it is essential to describe them here (Table 2.1).

Scientific research

This is a way of understanding the natural world by discovering laws of nature that (as yet) are hidden from us because (as yet) we have imperfect methods of investigation. It assumes there is 'truth' out there, which it is the task of researchers to uncover. Scientific research is deterministic and positivist. It sets out to be objective, to

Table 2.1   Four research traditions

	Scientific research	Survey research	Illuminative research	Action research
Examples	Randomised controlled trial, experimentation	Questionnaire, interview (schedules)	Observation, interview (open ended)	Observation, questionnaires, interviews
Scope	Physical world	Social world	Social world	Social world
Purposes	To identify truth, laws, to be applied to practice	To identify facts, test grand theories, to change practice	To identify opinions, to generate theory, to develop practice	Actions to improve practice through involvement of practitioners
Scale	Large	Large	Small	Local
Interest served	Technical	Practical	Practical	Emancipatory
Development metaphor	Moulding	Growth	Illumination	Empowerment

detach the researcher from the subject being researched – for fear of contamination of the findings or biasing the results.

The most common form of scientific investigation is the experiment, and in health care the 'gold standard' is the randomised controlled trial. Variables that might influence a phenomenon are identified, a few at a time are manipulated, the remainder are controlled. One group of subjects receives an intervention whilst another, which matches the first in all other respects, does not. Any subsequent difference is thus due to the intervention. Typically, the data are quantitative and are handled analytically, frequently utilising some form of statistical procedure. The outcome is evaluated in terms of its probability of occurring through chance.

So the purpose of scientific research is to discover value-free (that is objective) law-like (that is context-free) generalisations. In health care, its further purpose is to discover new knowledge that can be applied to practice.

Perhaps inevitably, scientific research makes a clear distinction between researchers and practitioners. More particularly, it places research and theory above practice, which by its very nature is held to be subjective and context-dependent. Scientific research aims to find out new things. It is competitive. Researchers want to 'get there first', to be the first to make the discovery, and this 'success' is recognised and reinforced (again typically in health care) by attaching the name of the discoverer to the discovery. Scientific research and professional fame go together.

Surveys

This form of research has strongly influenced most of our colleagues. It addresses social situations. A survey investigates observable facts and people's behaviour, but on a grand scale. A typical example is the public opinion poll which gathers data, often through the use of questionnaires or interview schedules, from large numbers of subjects so as to reduce the effects of variation and researcher bias.

In survey research the data are collected retrospectively, after the event has occurred (whilst much scientific research aims to be prospective). Survey data are often analysed statistically, though frequently descriptively (e.g. percentages), often utilising parametric techniques (for example, arithmetical means and standard deviations). The findings identify proportions, trends, groupings and so on, and test out already established theories which themselves are on a grand scale (for example, learning styles research) (see Coles, 1985).

So the aim of survey research is to 'find out what is happening', and through this to inform the people involved or responsible, either to confirm and maintain the actions already taken or to modify these in accordance with the research data.

As with the scientific tradition, survey researchers are experts in the methods they use and are thus different (and separate) from practitioners (though some practitioners undertake survey research). Nevertheless, survey research (like scientific research) remains separate from practice. Its findings must still be 'applied' to practice to bring about any change.

Illuminative research

This too investigates social phenomena but, unlike survey research, is most often small scale. This research attempts to shed light on the situations being studied (Parlett and Hamilton, 1972). Examples include research into what happens in an outpatients' clinic or during a patient–nurse interview. The intention is to illuminate the situation for those involved. It employs ethnographic methods (such as those used in anthropology). It observes and records, and often interviews the people involved. The data collected include people's perceptions, perspectives, and opinions of what is occurring as well as their views of their relationships with others in the situation.

This research is inevitably (perhaps essentially) subjective, and it uses this apparent weakness as one of its strengths. Researchers deliberately form a relationship with the people being researched (they might even become participant observers) so as to identify as closely as possible with the people whose views and opinions they are researching. The error involved in this approach is minimised through 'triangulation', by taking multiple perspectives on the situation, by employing more than one researcher and by utilising a number of data collection methods.

The findings are then interpreted (and this research is sometimes termed 'interpretative') by the researchers themselves since they are closest to the data collection process. Frequently illuminative research generates theory (rather than testing it) and thus identifies theory which is 'grounded' (Grundy, 1987) in the situation being researched.

Action research

This is also social research but differs from surveys and illuminative research in that it seeks deliberately to improve the situation being researched through direct action involving the participants. It employs data collection methods common to other forms of social research (for example observation, interviews and questionnaires) as the first stage of what has been called an action research cycle (Grundy, 1987). The data collected are then reflected upon by the researchers and participants. This leads to action planning so as to determine what should happen to improve the situation, and these actions once taken lead to further observation and data collection, thus recommencing the cycle.

The intention then of this research is action to improve, with the involvement of the participants. Terms such as empowerment and emancipation are often used to characterise this research process (Grundy, 1987).

These four research traditions then were known to our colleagues before they undertook this project, and they are commonly known to many health professionals. There are of course differences between them, in their purposes, their methods and their philosophical underpinnings. Yet they have certain features in common, and it is these that we wish to focus attention on here.

Research has come to be seen as objective, or (if that is difficult because of the methods used to collect data) as something which can be objectified through trying to ensure (in particular ways) that the data are not contaminated by the researcher and certainly not by the people (or situations) being researched.

So research is seen as (necessarily) separate from practice and researchers as (necessarily) different from practitioners. Indeed, researchers need to develop research skills which themselves are seen as technical in nature.

But more than this, research has come to be seen from the practitioners' viewpoint as something that others (outsiders, researchers) do to them. Researchers 'come in' and 'carry out' research. Then they 'go away' and work on the findings, and eventually 'come back' with the results. And perhaps worse, the researchers present practitioners with their conclusions (no matter how much this is disguised as 'negotiation' or 'consultation').

So the results of a research project are then to be 'applied' to practice. The conclusions of the research become the recommendations for action, which are to be taken up in practice in one form or another. Indeed, further projects are then undertaken to 'get research into practice'. This seems to hint at the difficulties (and frustrations) researchers have when practitioners (apparently stubbornly) refrain from doing (or refuse to do) what seems so obvious to the researchers.

References

Coles, C. R. (1985). Differences between conventional and problem-based learning curricula in their students' approaches to studying. *Medical Education*, **19**, 4308–4309.

Greenhalgh, T. (1996). Is my practice evidence-based? *British Medical Journal*, **313**, 957–958.

Grundy, S. (1987). *Curriculum: Product or Praxis?* The Falmer Press.

Kaplan, S. H., Greenfield, S. and Ware, J. E. (1989). Impact of the Doctor–Patient Relationship on the outcomes of Chronic Disease. In *Communicating with Medical Patients* (M. Stewart and D. Roter, eds.), pp. 228–245. Sage Publications.

Parlett, M. R. and Hamilton, D. (1972). *Evaluation as Illumination: a New Approach to the Study of Innovatory Programmes.* Occasional Paper 9, Centre for Research in the Educational Sciences.

Chapter 3

Seeing anew: understanding professional practice as artistry

Introduction

In the previous two chapters we have attempted to characterise the world of professional practice. In Chapter 1 we refer to professional work generally while in Chapter 2 we focus on the specific issues and problems in health care and to some extent also characterise the views of our colleagues who contribute to Part Two below. Thus, Chapter 1 represents the probable views of our likely readership and Chapter 2 shows the kinds of ideas our contributors held about practice in health care as this book began to be written.

In Chapter 1, then, we presented something of what it is to be a professional in the late twentieth century and described what seems to us to be the nature of professionalism as seen from within a range of professions today. We identified too some profound ironies which arise from some key paradoxes of professional practice today. For example, we noted the centrality of professional judgement to the work of a professional and yet the difficulty experienced by professionals in talking clearly about it. We would now add that problems arise in particular because, when professional judgement is being operated successfully, it is invisible and thus unable to be observed let alone measured either by outsiders or professionals themselves. Only when professionals make bad judgements is there a demand for accountability and then professionals' inability to explain it seems to compound the felony. We also noted the parallel point that professional activities require great expertise but that professionals, while they are able to act expertly, often cannot articulate what their expertise involves. This is especially a problem when professionals must pass on their expertise to others (that is, teach) and explore it further (that is, research).

The second chapter then showed how these generalisations become specific in health care and also illustrated the knock-on effects of these problems for health professionals in terms of their practice, their preparation for and development of it, and consequent views about ways of enquiring into it.

By contrast to the first two chapters, Chapter 3 provides alternative perspectives on professional practice and simultaneously indicates some of the views held by us as the editors of this work and the generators of this project. Chapter 4 then builds on this to look at the implications of these ideas for enquiring into practice, and for seeing practitioner research in a new way.

Intentions of this chapter

Our arguments in this chapter are essentially that professional practice is able to be characterised in terms of artistry and that this view brings with it a range of other new ways of seeing practice and theory, and uncovers a major obligation for professionals to try to understand better the *principles* (and not just the actions) on which their practice rests and to recognise fully and be able to articulate the nature of it. These arguments can be found in detail in Fish (in press), where the role of artist as someone who sees anew and shares that new vision with others is also explored.

Those parts of professional practice which seem routine or are merely about following procedures may be able to be dealt with for the purposes of accountability by collecting and supplying data for audit and individual performance review (IPR) as managerial tools. But, we argue here, professional practice contains a major element of artistry and this does not yield simple empirical evidence. We therefore believe that it is important for professionals to be able to reflect upon, articulate, refine and defend their practice. We believe that this is important not only in order to improve practice but also to enable the public better to understand that practice and, as a result, to adjust their expectations of professional practitioners. We also try to show why we believe that part of this enterprise of understanding professional practice and of recognising the artistry in it involves focusing upon one's own professional judgements and seeing one's individual practice within the broader context of the traditions of the practice of one's profession.

It will be apparent that our views as expressed here are in conflict with those we reported in the previous chapters which characterise the context in which we see professionals practising today. But, although we are apparently flying in the face of current ideas by calling for greater emphasis on and recognition of both professional artistry and professional judgement, we believe that there are very sound and long-standing arguments in theory as well as evidence in practice for the significance of both. These arguments are presented in greater detail in Fish (in press). In Chapters 3 and 4 here we consider writings which have helped us to see our thinking afresh and enabled us to understand the traditions of thought and of practice to which our ideas belong. In doing this we seek to offer readers some arguments that will help them in articulating the foundations of their own practices.

Professionalism as artistry

There is nothing new in claiming that professional practice in health care can be characterised as artistry. Medicine was originally regarded as an art and there is currently much discussion in nursing, occupational therapy and acupuncture about the artistry involved in their practices (see Fish, in press). But the significance of this issue seems to us to be deepening.

We believe that the health care professions of the late 1990s and those who work in them are tormented by two incompatible views of professionalism. Clear manifestations of both these views are visible – for those who look – in currently emerging approaches to professional development across health care. Understanding these is, we believe, the first step to seeing professional practice anew and to recognising the responsibilities that this new view brings with it.

On the one hand reflective practice (which, as we noted in Chapter 2, our contributors were well aware of even at the start of this project) is being hailed as the way forward in professions like nursing, where many professionals now treat it as a shibboleth, believing that it is a new term for thinking about one's practice which they have 'always done'. Yet, coincidentally, continuous quality improvement (CQI), and total quality management (TQM) have also become hot issues in health care as a whole (Berwick, 1996; Taylor, 1996) and there are demands that bureaucrats should impose system-wide procedures, such as protocols and guidelines, which will require professionals to follow rules and enable them apparently to stop thinking for themselves (see Fish, in press).

Beneath such conflicting initiatives, then, we suggest there lurk two different views of what a professional is and how a professional should behave, and these in turn are influenced by two very different sets of values. Following the work of Schön (1983 and 1987), we see these as the technical rational view of professionalism (which cashes out into a competency-based approach to practice which accepts the bureaucratic system-wide constraints of professionals) and the professional artistry view of professionalism (which, as we shall see, leads to a more serious form of reflective practice than is currently commonly found in health care).

It seems to us that the technical rational view is held broadly by the public (which includes the press and politicians but who are also the pool from which health care's clients and patients emerge). But, we would argue, professionals recognise that this view does not fit with their experience and that the professional artistry view represents ways of thinking about professional practice which those who know it from the inside recognise as more nearly what practice is actually like. Schön first drew attention to these views, and they were first published in this form in Fish (1991) and have been explored further by us, in Coles (1996, 1997) and in Fish (1995, 1996).

Two views: their overall notions of professional practice

The technical rational (TR) view of professionalism catches health care practice up into the late twentieth century behaviour of labelling everything in mechanistic terms. It views professional practice as a basic matter of delivering a service to clients through a pre-determined set of clear-cut routines and behaviours. The metaphor of 'delivery' has become so common that it appears as an unquestioned part of discussion in both health care and education. Yet some would point to the insidiousness with which the term – drawn from commercial and market-driven activities like getting the newspapers, milk and bread to customers' doorsteps – has gained acceptance for describing the activity of working with patients/clients. Its acceptance shows just how far members of the public and we as professionals have been seduced by the idea that technology and business are a paradigm of all useful human activity. And its most pernicious influence is its penetration of our subconscious with the idea that the 'deliverer' (the professional) is someone who must not tamper with the goods (the package) he or she is delivering, but is simply an agent for conveying safely something created by one body to another. The term 'delivery' then is thus both a major means to, and a key signal of, the success of the downgrading of professionalism, via a TR view of it. Indeed, for education Carr and Hartnett (1996) demonstrate how deep these issues go by tracing in detail the deintellectualisation of policy in relation to that profession. Some strong parallels between what has happened in education and in health care can be deduced from their work.

The TR approach to health care, of prescribing and proscribing all the practitioner's activities, is flagged as being able to cut down considerably the risks incurred when professionals make more of their own decisions. Here the ever-present threat from accountability has been allowed to push the practitioner into such a defensive frame of mind that he or she is constantly in a 'no-win position', where both to act and not to act is equally likely to invite litigation, and where it is only possible to defend activities which come within the pre-specified rules. And it assumes that practice is a relatively simple interaction in which the practitioner gives and patients and clients receive, and which can be perfected.

By contrast, those who espouse a professional artistry (PA) view of professionalism believe that the TR view is a deficit view of professionals and denies the real character of both professionalism and practice. They argue that far from being simple and predictable, professional practice involves a more complex and less certain 'real world' in which, daily, the professional is involved in making many complex decisions, relying on a mixture of professional judgement, intuition and common sense, and that these activities are not able to be set down in absolute routines, or be made visible in simple terms, and certainly are not able to be measured, and which because of this are extremely difficult to teach and to research.

Their view of the activities of a professional

The TR view then, characterises professional activities as essentially able to be pre-specified and susceptible to being broken down into their component parts. Such parts are all regarded as 'skills' and are thus viewed as being able to be mastered. The TR view further regards being a professional as being essentially efficient in 'the' skills, and submissive in harnessing them to carry out other people's decisions. Such skills, it is assumed, can be listed beforehand, and are now commonly referred to as competencies, or, sometimes, 'performance outcomes'. The identification of these skills, which are superficially reassuring in their ability to be seen and measured, make professional accountability superficially easy. Thus, competencies or 'outcomes' have for some time now dominated many courses of preparation for professional practice and are currently proposed as the basis for university courses and for staff development in the professions. In this way the technical rational view of professionalism and the competency-based approach to practice is rapidly gaining ground as the only view.

The PA view, by major contrast, sees behaving professionally as being concerned with both means and ends. Here, professional activity is more akin to artistry, where only the *principles* can be pre-determined and practitioners may in practice and for good reason need to choose to go beyond them, just as, say, good artists often go beyond or break artistic conventions in order to achieve an important effect. Thus, in this view, practitioners are broadly autonomous, making their own decisions about their actions and the moral bases of those actions (for which, of course, they are accountable). In the PA view, the *activities* of the professional cannot be pre-specified, just as a painter cannot tell you what the picture he or she is creating will be like until it is finished.

Thus, too, the characteristics of 'good practice' are regarded as context specific because, again like the artist, the professional has to harness on the spot professional judgement as to what to do since every situation is to some extent unique. Further, the PA view recognises that there are many components of professional activity (just as there are many things involved in artistic activity) and not all of them are able to be distinguished one from another, and some of them are tacit. There will, of course, in any piece of professional practice be of necessity routine and unreflecting parts of daily professional life, but loss of sight of fundamental principles on which one has come to believe that one's practice should be founded is (to adapt Golby, 1993, p. 5) at once a loss of professionalism. In this model, then, the professional is not less accountable, but is in fact accountable for more – for skills of course, but also for much more important moral and ethical matters that underpin their decision-making and judgement. Here, to be professional is to be morally answerable for all of one's conduct, and for one's conduct as a whole, not just for parts of it.

But this brings with it the problem of how to render visible the invisible, and how to view the whole not just the parts. How can one 'see' the moral basis of one's judgement? Such a problem is acute when the invisible is – as we shall argue professional judgement indeed is – the very centre and the distinguishing mark of one's professionalism.

Our contention is that it can be made visible by articulating one's practice in full, that is, articulating not merely the surface fact, the observable 'doing' of professional practice, but the invisible depths below it. We also believe that if professional practice is akin to art, it is entirely appropriate in capturing and investigating professional activities to draw upon artistic means of investigation and of expression, because art is concerned with conveying the subtleties and ineffable aspects of life, and does so without first needing to attempt to atomise it into parts (see Fish, in press). The attempt to think about practice is sometimes characterised as 'reflective practice', but it is not often seen as rigorous, and in our experience until now it has rarely involved the serious level of enquiry and a deep consideration of the artistry of the professional that we are arguing for.

Their views about professional expertise

Thus, the TR view believes in the centrality of rules, schedules, prescriptions, whereas the PA view believes that, as in the work of the artist, so in the work of a professional, practice starts where the rules fade (because the rules rarely fit real practice). Thus, the PA view relies on frameworks and rules of thumb, rather than rules. The TR view emphasises diagnosis, analysis, and efficient systems. It believes in detailed job specifications, protocols and guidelines, that is, in being able to analyse a professional role down to the last detail. The PA view by contrast, believes instead in interpretation of details, acknowledges the inevitable subjectivity of setting them down, and comes to an understanding of professional activities by means of appreciation (as in the critical appreciation of art and music). It wishes to encourage not narrow efficiency but creativity and the right to be wrong. The TR model assumes that knowledge is permanent, able to be totally mastered, and is thus worth attempting to master. The PA view is that knowledge is temporary, dynamic and problematic, and that it is more useful to know processes than to know facts.

Their views of professional practice

The professional artistry approach sees professional practice as complex. Just as a painting, a poem or a piece of music demands a response to its entirety which would not be satisfied only by analysing it technically into its component parts, so professional practice needs to be understood holistically. This inevitably raises deep questions about what is involved in professional expertise seen as artistry. The following might well be raised.

- How is practice (which is artistic in nature) learnt and how can it be improved?
- How far is self-knowledge significant?
- In the exercise of artistry, how can we come to understand better the thought and action involved?
- How can we investigate artistry in ways that aid our understanding of it?

By comparison, those who subscribe to the TR view would argue that professional practice need not be that complex, has for too long been surrounded by a mystique and has now advanced to the point where goals can be set by society for professionals whose role is purely instrumental. For example they might point to the very language of health care today, including 'clinical guidelines; clinical outcomes; health outcome individualisation; health technology assessment [which] all form part of NHS (National Health Service) strategies for improving the effectiveness of the service it provides'

(Culshaw, 1995, p. 323). They would argue that this shows that the professional's role can indeed be analysed technically and rationally in terms of activities and skills (though in the end this can lead to an obsessive intention to tie things down further and further in the inevitably vain attempt to try to cater for all eventualities).

Their views about how to improve practice

The TR view of professional development sees it as a simple matter of providing skills training. Practice, in TR terms, is easily learnt. But the PA view sees the TR approach as unable to meet the real situations of practice which is messy, unpredictable, unexpected. The PA view recognises the importance in practitioners of the artistic ability to improvise (an ability often *diminished* by training and routine). Also, because practice is rapidly changing, it requires the practitioner autonomously to be able to refine and update his or her expertise 'on the hoof', which is what reflective practice is about (and what professional development should be about) and which those who subscribe to this view would argue is more cost effective than endlessly changing the system. Here, to improve practice is to treat it more holistically, to work to understand its complexities, and to look carefully at one's actions and theories as one works and, subsequently, to challenge them with ideas from other perspectives, and to seek to improve and refine practice and its underlying theory. Here, the professional is working towards increased competence (but not towards acquired competencies, see Fish, 1996). Those committed to the TR view, however, would argue that this is all too woolly (because it admits of less certainty). Further, it does not please politicians (who represent professional views to the public in simplistic terms because they do not fully understand the complexities of professional practice and do not share the values and perspectives of professionals). Politicians undervalue the professional artistry view of practice and the reflective practitioner approach that it brings with it because its fruits may show up less clearly in the short term since it emphasises aspects that are not simple, visible behaviours. But in fact, as we argue throughout this book and demonstrate in our colleagues' contributions to Part Two, it offers in the long term scope for deeper-rooted improvements, which are owned by the professional.

Their views about theory

But it is, perhaps, in its views about theory that the TR model is most highly specific and – for us – the most suspect. It sees theory as 'Formal Theory' produced by researchers (who, as we noted in Chapter 2, stand apart from the practitioners). This formal theory is to be learnt and then applied to practice. It regards practice as an arena in which to demonstrate previously worked-out theory. By contrast, the PA view is that theory is implicit in (underlies) all action, that (as for the artist) both action and theory are developed *in practice*. This means that refining practice involves unearthing the theories on which that practice is founded and that formal theory aids the development of practice by challenging and extending the practitioner's understandings. This view (that with the help of reflection theory emerges *from* practice) enables the professional to examine and develop personal theory as it arises from that practice. Such personal theory is implicit in all action but needs to be unearthed from beneath it in order to be acknowledged, understood and used to inform decisions about later action. It is also able to be refined by recourse to further practice and to the wider view of theory offered by other theorists and researchers.

The TR view, then, emphasises the 'known', and is in tune with present trends in that it celebrates certainty and hard evidence. By contrast the PA view recognises the value of uncertainty, humility and critical scepticism and is willing to accept the notion of mystery within human activity. It regards the activity of the professional as not entirely able to be analysed down to the last atom, even if the routinised craft skills on which artistry is based are able to be specified. It regards professional practitioners as eternal seekers rather than 'knowers'. It sees the activities of the professional as mainly open capacities which by definition are not able to be mastered. (The test of an open capacity is that the learner can take steps which he has not been taught to take, which in some measure would surprise the teacher and perhaps the learner.)

The professional artistry view, then, sees professional practice as an art in which risks are inevitable if there is to be any creativity, where learning to do is only achieved by engaging in doing and reflecting upon the doing, and where improvisation, enquiry into action and resulting insight by those involved in it generate a major knowledge base.

This idea goes back to Greek thought where the term 'praxis' (which approximates to the kind of professional practices we are describing) is, as Aristotle argued, action in which the end product is not an object but is the realisation of morally worthwhile good (see, for example, Carr, 1995). Thus, in health care for instance, the good that practitioners seek is health and perhaps education (and the health care educator is certainly concerned with both 'goods'). Such good cannot be *made* outside the practice and then delivered to it, but can only be done within it. That is, the ends cannot be absolutely designed in advance of engaging in the practice. Although they might be *formulated* in theory, they are not fixed, but are mutable and develop as the practice develops. And they are only intelligible in terms of the traditions of good (health and education) which are being practised. As we show in Parts Two and Three, professional judgement is at the centre of this.

These ideas have profound significance for *preparation* for practice in health care at all levels from undergraduate (pre-registration) training, in learning to carry out day-to-day work in practical situations, through to life-long professional development itself.

The notion that the details of practice cannot be pre-determined fiercely challenges the orthodox assumption that health care practitioners need to be well prepared for practice by being trained in routines and given knowledge to apply in situ. In fact, ironically, such routines, which are designed to provide a good basis for practice, can be very dangerous for patients and undesirable for practitioners. Routines can obscure the realities of real practice for and with the individual patients. Those who see their practice only through the veil of such routines, will only *perceive* it as routine – even when it is not so. Learning routines and applicatory knowledge is also undesirable for practitioners because the 'auto pilot' nature of routine and the application of knowledge obliterates the detail from which practitioners could learn by thinking about their practice both during it and afterwards. The need for practitioners in health care to appear as experts who are 'unshakeable', then, is not best provided for by preparing *for* practice, by being equipped with pre-determined routines. It is better met by being prepared *to* practise, by being alerted to the messy and complex nature of practice, by treating the knowledge one has as adaptable, and by being made conscious of principles upon which one's practice is based and of the need to use these to 'make meaning' in the particular situation. It is about being prepared to meet and work with the unexpected.

It is for this reason that it is not possible in heath care and education to train student practitioners in all they need to operate their practice. And it never will be. It is not that we currently lack the right knowledge and technology to train practitioners in 'the right procedures', and that we shall 'crack' this in time. The entire idea is a chimera. It may be true in terms of scientific and technical knowledge that when we have more factual knowledge we shall be able to put it into practice and thus improve our end product. But that is not true of practice (or praxis), as all practitioners really know at heart. Here, the improvement of practice itself is an improvement of *understanding* and comes as part of the doing and the reflection upon it. Improvement of practice is entirely in the hands of the practitioner.

Their views about quality

Each model also gives rise to a particular view of quality. The TR model speaks in the language of quality assurance and control. It places emphasis upon visible performance. It seeks to test and measure these, believing that technical performance is all-important. Thus the model is behaviourist, emphasises fixed standards, controls professional practice via inspection and IPR, and believes that change can be imposed from outside the profession and that quality is measurable. It is characterised by 'a centralist surveillance of standards' (Carr and Hartnett, 1996, p. 176). Ironically though, it holds the professional practitioner accountable only for his or her *technical* expertise. This is because it unconsciously but inevitably denies the existence of professional judgement and a moral dimension to professional practice (or perhaps believes that it is only a matter of time before it is expressed in simplified procedures as clinical reasoning already is). It also has the effect of demotivating the professional by reducing the challenge that autonomy offers, and turning practice into a factory-like monotony and the practitioner into a delivery agent.

By contrast, the PA view sees that there is more to professional practice than its surface and visible features, more to the whole than the sum of the parts, more to competence than an accumulation of competencies. It believes in the unavoidable significance of professional judgements in professional practice, holds that the most easily measurable is often also the most trivial, and that issues involving moral complexities are never resolved by resort to empiricism.

Most importantly, the PA view wishes to harness investigation, reflection and deliberation (and, we would add, appreciation) in order to enable professionals to develop their own insights from inside their own practice. It holds that this is a better means of staff development than change imposed from without. In short, it believes that quality comes from deepening insight into one's own values, priorities, actions. Under this model it is possible (and necessary) to talk about wide professional answerability rather than narrow technical accountability. This makes professionals responsible for the moral dimensions of professional action, and for reflecting upon, investigating and refining their own practice. It enables practitioners to own their practice and to enjoy improving it.

Table 3.1 offers a summary of the points in our argument so far.

Some conclusions about professional practice

We reject the technical rational view of 'health care delivery' because it makes the following assumptions:

- that quality health care practice is achieved only through the strict adherence to well thought out (and evidence-based) guidelines and protocols;
- that health professionals (especially junior ones, as lower status professionals) are not capable of making judgements (or should not be expected to);
- that professional judgements are dangerous departures from established procedures because they allow too much variability in situations that require to be controlled.

We believe too that the technical rational approach:

- ignores the existence of the judgements that all health professionals take all the time;
- denies the importance of people making these judgements quite appropriately in delivering high quality health care;

Table 3.1   Two views of professional practice

The technical rational (TR) view	The professional artistry (PA) view
Follows rules, laws, routines and prescriptions	Starts where rules fade, sees patterns, frameworks
Uses diagnosis, analysis	Uses interpretation/appreciation
Wants efficient systems	Wants creativity and room to be wrong
Sees knowledge as graspable, permanent	Knowledge is temporary, dynamic, problematic
Theory is applied to practice	Theory emerges from practice
Visible performance is central	There is more to it than surface features
Setting out and testing for basic competency is vital	There is more to it than the sum of the parts
Technical expertise is all	Professional judgement counts
Sees professional activities as masterable	Sees mystery at the heart of professional activities
Emphasises the known	Embraces uncertainty
Standards must be fixed Standards are measurable and must be controlled	That which is most easily fixed and measurable is also often trivial – professionals should be trusted
Emphasises assessment, IPR, inspection, accreditation	Emphasises investigation, reflection, deliberation
Change must be managed from outside	Professionals can develop from inside
Quality is really about the quantity of that which is easily measurable	Quality comes from deepening insight into one's values, priorities, actions
Technical accountability	Professionals answerability
This is training	This is education
It takes the instrumental view	It sees education as intrinsically worthwhile

Source: This table was first published in this form in Fish, D. (1995). *Quality Mentoring for Student Teachers: A Principled Approach to Practice*. David Fulton, p. 43.

- fails to help health professionals make explicit the basis of their judgements;
- fails to enable health professionals to develop and refine their professional judgements.

But a word of caution. The professional artistry view does not refute the value of skills. It merely wishes to see their significance within a broader focus. Nor does it assume that all the judgements that professionals make are appropriate, or that departing from clinical guidelines on a health professional's whim will inevitably lead to better health care. On the contrary, professional artistry holds professionals responsible for their actions and recognises that the quality of health care rests on the appropriateness of the judgements made. However, it suggests that these judgements are often made intuitively and inevitably on very little explicit information, and that health professionals rarely have the opportunity of making their judgements explicit or to discuss, debate and critically appreciate them. Indeed our experience is that getting health professionals to articulate their intuitive judgements is actually quite difficult (and that it is even more difficult to get them to make the time to do so).

A professional artistry view of professionalism recognises, then, the professional responsibility (moral and ethical as well as practical) that lies behind the making of judgements. We believe that a technical rational view of professional action diminishes a health care worker's professionalism, where a professional artistry view enhances that professionalism.

We know professionals who agree with this but find the PA view hard to defend because they are not familiar with these arguments. We are also aware that some professionals are afraid that the PA approach is too woolly, subjective, temporary and unable to be taught, and that those trained in the TR view appear to 'know more'.

This book is devoted to providing health care professionals with a basis for weighing these arguments. It attempts to demonstrate that serious reflective practice involves at least as much rigour as any other form of enquiry. And it seeks to illustrate how in unearthing and discovering the hidden treasures of their professional judgements, practitioners can enrich their professional lives and as a consequence can improve the quality of the lives of those for whom they care.

For the professional, as for the artist, such an unearthing of the basis of one's practice needs, however, to be informed by an understanding of the nature of that practice generally and of the relationship of practice to theory. The following is an attempt to set out our understanding of these matters in respect of professional practice itself. A basis for understanding practice and theory in terms of artistry will emerge in Part Three and can also be found in Fish (1998). First, however, we need to clarify the term 'professional

practice' itself and to highlight an important d
two very different usages of it.

Professional practice: two usages

The term 'professional practice' can refer to the *indi*   *y*
or activities of a single practitioner and also to wh. Golby has
called a 'whole tradition in which particular activities are related
together as part of a social project or mission' (Golby, 1993, p. 4).
For education, he notes, the social project is the promotion of
knowledge, just as for the legal profession it is justice and for the
medical profession it is health. For the artist too, tradition is very
important (see Langford, 1985 and Fish, in press).

Individual activities in professional practice, as Golby (1981)
argues, are best understood from within the tradition of professional practice to which they are related. They are at best temporary (can never be fully solved) and situation specific. They are
essentially contestable (because value-related) and have a moral
dimension. Indeed, learning to practise in a profession is an open
capacity, cannot be mastered and goes on being refined for ever.
Arguably there is a major onus on those who teach courses of
preparation for professional practice to demonstrate this and to
reveal in *their* practice its implications.

Thus, learning to become a professional – or an artist – (which
continues throughout a professional's career) is 'a matter of coming
ever more fully into membership of a tradition of practice' and, 'at
its maturity it is a matter of taking part in more fully shaping
practice for the future'. This involves understanding the inherited
traditions of a profession (and/or of the preparation to enter that
profession), and considering critically and practically their present
relevance (see Golby, 1993, p. 8, and Fish, 1995, pp. 73–74).

We are now in a position to summarise our views about the
nature of professional practice in its profession-wide sense.

The nature of professional practice: a summary

The following summarises the ideas about professional practice
which we would wish to argue for.

e see professional practice as having the nature of artistry.

- We recognise the central place of professional judgement in professional practice and the *raison d'être* of professionalism as resting upon it.
- We see practice (rather than theory) as of prime significance and as a proper starting point for professional preparation and development.
- We believe that professional knowledge is created in and during practice.
- We see such knowledge as emerging from critical reflection on, enquiry into and deliberation about experience.
- We believe (following Eraut, 1994) that it is informed by formal knowledge which is transformed in practice to become personal knowledge.
- We acknowledge practice and theory as developing reflexively together.
- We value the processes of theorising from practice as central to reflection and deliberation.
- We see professional development as a process of changing people by educating them rather than by changing systems and training people to adapt to them – we see it as a process of evolving change from within rather than imposing change from without.

Such ideas challenge the notions about professional practice that some practitioners and most of the public have held routinely (and therefore unexamined) for many years. These notions are as follows:

- that theory is intrinsically more valuable than practice and that practice is merely a vehicle for putting into operation Formal Theory;
- that theory can be applied to practice, practice is subsidiary to the theory, and that practitioners are merely the operators of someone else's theory;
- that health care professionals are – or should be – absolute experts in terms of their *health care knowledge* and that trust of the public in the professional should rest on this alone;
- that not being theorists, 'practitioners are poorly informed about practice even though they know it from the inside' (Carr, 1995, p. 10).

As we pointed out in Chapter 1, professional people are under siege in many respects. Not least of their problems is the loss of trust in them by society. Relationships between professionals and clients or patients have traditionally been trusting ones. To take advantage of professional services was inevitably to accept that professionals would do what they could and that they would maintain confidentiality. Now the very basis of that trust is under challenge and the fiduciary relationship has become eroded. This loss of trust has been nurtured by the prevailing climate of technical rationalism which demystifies professionalism, but which leaves nothing in its place. There is thus a certain irony in the way health care is now provided (in the United Kingdom) through the creation of hospital Trusts. The term is being used here, presumably, in the sense of financial resources being entrusted to a group of people who must provide sound stewardship of it. But, ironically, this is quite different from any trust (which society might accord to the people running Trusts) that they will provide effective health care.

All these ideas bring with them the inevitable assumptions that in courses of professional preparation formal theory and specialist knowledge must come first, that they ought to be the basis for professional development and research, and that practice only really gains its significance in applicatory relationship to Formal Theory and as demonstrated by absolute expertise.

They also support the common myth that theory is a quite separate activity from practice. But this so called 'theory–practice gap' is actually an artefact of the technical rational view of professional education. It can only be thought to exist where there is a belief that there is a clear separation of academic knowledge from practical knowledge, of formal theory from personal theory.

The PA approach, with its emphasis on a holistic view of practice, could not conceive of such a separation of theory and practice. Here, practice is the starting point for understanding theory. Hence the notion that practice rather than theory is of prime significance for the professional practitioner just as it is for the working artist. That is, practice is a reference point. It enables us both to give meaning to our ideas as they emerge from practice and to set the ideas which interest us back into context. In all this, the refinement of practice is the most important end of our endeavours.

However, this does not deny or reduce the importance to practitioners of theory. Indeed, we believe that it is important for practitioners to recognise that theory underpins their practice, that they are theorists and that they can or should work at theorising their practice. We agree with Eraut that formal knowledge (knowledge formulated outside practice) is not really able to be directly applied in practice but rather, must be *transformed* by the practitioner and must become incorporated into the practitioner's personal knowledge if that knowledge is to inform the practitioner's practice. In a very real sense professionals *create* professional knowledge in their practice (see Eraut, 1994, p. 43). For these reasons we must now turn to theory, and through that to consider in Chapter 4 what research means in the context of professional practice.

Theories and theorising: some definitions

The work of Smith brings a fresh and useful perspective in helping us to clarify both what we mean by theory and what theorising – a process of investigation – can offer a professional practitioner. Within this broad view of theory, Smith distinguishes between reflective (personal) theory and formal (public) theory, and he makes the point that both kinds of theory can be practice-focused (Smith, 1992, p. 393). He argues that there is often too *little* theorising in professional education rather than too much and adds:

> For it is where there is insufficient critical, analytical thinking that the dreary orthodoxies take root and the ghosts of dead theories roam unchecked. Unless [professional practitioners] have sufficient understanding of the philosophies that are *presupposed* by what is taken as evidence, the scope of their reflectivity and thus their capacity for change is limited from the outset, and they are condemned to remain second-class citizens in the world of ideas. (Smith, 1992, p. 391)

Theorising practice involves revealing – in a controlled and balanced way – the depth of thought and feeling lying beneath our actions. That is, it involves recognising the wellsprings of our judgements, decisions, reasoning and actions, our beliefs, assumptions, values and theories. It includes recognising honestly the *results* within our practice of our assumptions, our reasoning, values, beliefs, judgements and action, and it involves identifying the problematic, the contestable, the dilemmas endemic to our practice. That is why we talk of it as a far more serious form of reflection than is usually implied by the word. We have more to say about it in respect of the processes it involves at the end of this chapter and again in the final section (Part Four) of this book.

Smith usefully recommends the term 'reflective theory' for such activities, perhaps because they involve the practitioner in standing back from practice (rather like an artist from the easel) and scrutinising what he or she is doing and examining the presuppositions and assumptions that he or she has made. (This is perhaps more often called **personal theory**.) Within the broad category of personal theory, Argyris and Schön long ago offered us the notion of **'espoused theory'** to denote theory which we say we hold and which we believe should shape our actions, and **'theory-in-use'** for those ideas that actually can be deduced from our actions because they actually inform, shape and explain them (Argyris and Schön, 1974, pp. 6–7). And as Tripp suggests, there is indeed an interesting gap here, not between theory and practice but rather between theory and theory, because everyone who looks can find interesting examples in their practice of a difference between what they say they (or others) should do, and what they actually do (Tripp, 1993, p. 147). This itself can offer a useful focus in trying to understand better and thence refine professional practice.

By contrast to this 'personal' theory, we would want to use the term **formal theory** for the results of processes Smith describes as:

> a more thorough-going scrutiny in which our ideas are challenged by other people, in which we read books and test our thinking against the ideas to be found in them, where we acquire a historical perspective, [and] wrestle with quite fundamental concepts... (Smith, 1992, p. 392)

He notes the 'near impossibility' of working at this without the support of higher education resources including staff. He adds that the significance of the nature and role of reflective and formal theory, 'is nothing less than the question of whether a profession is to be a properly *rational* enterprise or not'. (This is of course quite different from 'technical rational'.)

He suggests and then explores the following key tasks for reflective and formal theory in professional education, which he argues are student practitioners' entitlement, which we argue is every practitioner's entitlement and which we have summarised as follows:

- to challenge implicit theory already in practitioners' thinking;
- to show practitioners that ideas about and the activities of practice can be otherwise;
- to develop a sense of professional education (by examining ideas, metaphors, formulating a defensible personal theory of professional practice);
- to create an intelligent profession (accustomed to reading thoughtful and demanding books);
- to make professional practice interesting (to turn the potentially confusing and internally contestable into something intrinsically interesting – and unthreatening) (Smith, 1992, p. 392).

Clarifying the relationship of practice and theory

All of this leads us to offer the formal theoretical foundations of our view of the overall relationship between theory and practice before we finally look at what is involved in theorising practice. Here we have chosen to cite the work of Aristotle (through the work of Carr) as a major source because we see in it the most fundamental and persuasive of arguments about the relationship of theory and practice.

Practitioners tend to shy away from theory. They see it as failing to answer the questions it was supposed to resolve and even failing to agree the questions (see Carr and Hartnett, 1996, p. 7). They see theories as something other people have. And they see theory as unvalued by public and government alike, not recognising perhaps that such a downgrading of theory is a form of downgrading professions themselves. All this tends to leave practitioners with an uncomfortable feeling that they ought one day to sort out their views. And the result of this is that they work on the basis of unexamined views about theory – and therefore about practice!

At base, practitioners' unexamined views about professional practice often fall into two parts – their public view (supported by The Public) that theory is important and must somehow structure practice, and the private view that in their day-to-day activities of practice theory is actually less important and seems to have little real impact. If pressed to consider these two views further they often take refuge in talking of a gap between theory and practice or conversely argue that theory is mysteriously related to practice in some way practitioners have not yet fathomed (or do not have the time to fathom because they are too busy getting on with their practice). Such views are deep-seated and emerge in practice in a number of ways which themselves are rarely challenged. For example, several of our contributors clearly felt guilty when not turning first to a literature search and survey as the starting point for their research for this book, and many of them asked at different times for help with 'The Theory'. Others felt that the theorising they were undertaking was valuable but took rather a long time and by implication took them away from what they should have been doing. The following arguments provide a way of refuting these ideas.

The argument for a holistic view of practice and theory

As Carr illustrates, one or even several false and competing ideas and arguments about the relationship between theory and practice lie beneath many of the discussions about them and distort our understanding of them.

The argument that there is a gap between theory and practice arises from three basic ideas. For some, practice is theory-guided, for some practice is opposed to theory and for others practice is independent of theory. Carr (1995, pp. 60–73) offers a clear exposition of the reasons why each of these three ideas about practice are of themselves individually inadequate for determining how the concept of practice should be understood. During the course of this he also highlights the illogicality of those who argue that practice is somehow less important (and more messy) than theory. Readers are directed to the work of Carr (1995) for the finer details of his argument since what follows cannot do justice to it but offers only the gist.

In setting out his long but in our view important argument, Carr shows that it is unhelpful to define practice as theory-guided (that is, which both *presupposes* that practice has a conceptual framework and that external theory guides its processes) since action in the work of practitioners often quickly moves into areas where there is no direct theory to tell them what to do.

Furthermore, Carr points out, this idea (that practice, rather than being opposed to theory, is theory-guided) is unhelpful also because it suggests that practice is guided by theory *alone* which clearly is not true either, as a moment's thought about one's own practice would demonstrate. Thus, practice is not a *pure* version of theorising.

It is also unsatisfactory to define practice in contradistinction to theory, as if practice were everything that theory is not. This view is held by those who believe that theory is abstract and not located in place and time whereas practice is concrete and is context-related. But clearly, as Carr points out, this is too simplistic. Some problems of practice are more general and abstract than others and some call for immediate action which is actually based upon timeless questions that have always been debated by philosophers.

Yet to suggest that practice is entirely independent of thoery is to imply that there is no reasoning which guides it, no beliefs and values which drive it. This too is clearly untrue since many actions are carefully considered.

Carr then demonstrates that the opposition of practice to theory, the dependence of practice on theory and the independence of practice from theory are, in fact, all necessary features of practice but that alone each account offers a one-sided view – an incomplete analysis of practice.

He points out that it is a false assumption that the *meaning* of practice can only be determined by clarifying how it relates to theory, so that in order to understand what a practice is, it is always necessary to understand this relationship. (An example would be that most practising Christians are quite unable to explain the finer points of theology, and that being a practising Christian is not dependent on this.) This means that we can claim to understand what a practice involves even when we cannot explain how it relates to theory. This is just as well since some people (including ourselves) believe that we shall never totally understand practice and this allows us to discuss practice with a more open and comfortable acknowledgement of our incomplete picture of it. It also gives the lie to the notion that we can in a simple way 'apply theory to practice', and shows from a logical point of view (as well as from an empirical one) that we are unlikely ever to establish practice as entirely evidence-based.

As Carr, referring to Aristotle, shows then, knowledge of general theories is never enough to determine fully what the practitioner will do. What to do must be decided on the spot in the specific situation as part of the action. And this drawing upon principles and the simultaneous creating of the action in situ refine each other as they are being operated. And so theory cannot alone determine practice. Instead, it needs to be considered in respect of and in relationship to particular circumstances.

Thus Carr shows that 'understanding and applying principles are not ... two separate processes but mutually constitutive elements in the continuous dialectical reconstruction of knowledge and action' (Carr, 1995, p. 69). Such a reconstruction or transformation is often referred to as 'theorising practice'.

Theorising practice

It is by being theorised that practice gains its meaning. That is why theorising their practice is such an important activity for practitioners. The processes it draws upon include the analytical, interpretative and appreciative viewing and reviewing of the actions of practice in the wider context of the history and traditions of professional practice and in terms of the political, social and moral dimensions of the actions taken. This must be done in order to make more sense of them than appears on the surface. The notion of the extended professional, as described by Hoyle (1974) and developed by Stenhouse, was seen in just such terms as one who:

- viewed his or her work in the wider context;
- is concerned to link theory and practice;
- is committed to systematic questioning of professional practice as a basis for development;
- has a commitment and the ability to study his or her own professional practice;
- is concerned to question and test theory in practice by the use of those skills;
- is ready to allow others to observe his or her work and to discuss it with them on an open and honest basis. (Paraphrased from Stenhouse, 1975, pp. 143–144)

In this sense the familiar cry of what Hoyle calls 'restricted professionals' in reference to theorising and reflection that they 'do it all the time', is clearly not true. Such theorising must be systematic and publicly conducted, and, as our contributors found, is hard work and often uncomfortable – but then real learning is often like that.

Theorising, then, is an active uncovering of the thought, assumptions, beliefs and values that lie beneath practice, and it must be publicly carried out. The relationship between theory and practice must be understood in terms of the public not the private sphere. The professional is concerned for the public and not the private good. Collaboration in such enterprises is often important, and certainly our contributors grew to recognise the importance of their group experiences and shared explorations. That is why, too, research must have a public audience. Also, public theoretical knowledge has a different relationship to action from private knowledge. Theoretical knowledge, then, is mediated through the minds of individuals and through public processes in which actions come to be understood as practices, and whose meaning and significance is shared in groups – even communities. This is why talking of 'reflecting on practice' as if it were an armchair activity – a matter of thinking privately about one's actions in one's day-to-day work – is a travesty of the much more important activity we hope to demonstrate in this book.

The reasons why practitioners need to share their theorising about practice are explained by Kemmis. He makes the point that knowledge becomes theory by being tested, justified and sustained through debate in the public sphere. Theorising thus establishes agreements and disagreements between the new knowledge and what others know, by its reconciliation with what others have already contributed to the common stock of knowledge and thus it is given a place in the public realm of knowledge (Kemmis, 1995, p. 15).

Such theorising is a more major part of the investigation of (or 'research into') practice than is commonly realised as we shall try to demonstrate in the following chapter which will also act as an introduction to our colleagues' work.

References

Argyris, C. and Schön, D. (1974). *Theory in Practice: Increasing Professional Effectiveness*. Jossey-Bass.

Berwick, D. M. (1996). A primer on leading the improvement of systems. *British Medical Journal*, **312**, 619–622.

Carr, W. (1995). *For Education: Towards Critical Educational Enquiry.* Open University Press.

Carr, W. and Hartnett, A. (1996). *Education and the Struggle for Democracy: the Politics of Educational Ideas.* Open University Press.

Coles, C. (1996). Approaching professional development. *Journal of Continuing Education in the Health Professions*, 16, 152–158.

Coles, C. (1997). Training and the process of professional development. In *The Cambridge Handbook of Psychology, Health and Medicine* (A. Baum, C. McMannis, S. Newman *et al.* eds.), pp. 325–328. Cambridge University Press.

Culshaw, H. (1995). Evidence-based practice for sale? *British Journal of Occupational Therapy*, 58, 233.

Eraut, M. (1994). *Developing Professional Knowledge and Competence.* Falmer Press.

Fish, D. (1991). But can you prove it? Quality assurance and the reflective practitioner. *Assessment and Evaluation in Higher Education*, 16, 22–36.

Fish, D. (1995). *Quality Mentoring for Student Teachers: a Principled Approach to Practice.* David Fulton.

Fish, D. (1996). Competence: spelling out the problem. *Journal of Teacher Development*, 5, 58.

Fish, D. *Appreciating Practice in the Caring Professions: Re-focusing Professional Development and Practitioner Research.* Butterworth–Heinemann. In press.

Golby, M. (1981). Practice and theory. In *Rethinking Curriculum Studies* (M. Lawn and L. Barton, eds.), pp. 214–236. Croom Helm.

Golby, M. (ed.) (1993). Editorial comments. *Reflective Professional Practice: A Reader.* (Course 124 Papers for MEd students at Exeter University) Fair Way Publications.

Hoyle, E. (1974). Professionality, professionalism and the control of teaching. *London Educational Review*, 3, 13–18.

Kemmis, S. (1995). Prologue: theorising educational practice. In *For Education: Towards Critical Educational Enquiry* (W. Carr, ed.), pp. 1–17. Open University Press.

Langford, G. (1985). *Education, Persons and Society: a Philosophical Enquiry.* Macmillan.

Schön, D. (1983). *The Reflective Practitioner.* Basic Books.

Schön, D. (1987). *Educating the Reflective Practitioner.* Jossey-Bass.

Smith, R. (1992). Theory: an entitlement to understanding. *Cambridge Journal of Education*, 22, 387–398.

Stenhouse, L. (1975). *An Introduction to Curriculum Research and Development.* Heinemann.

Taylor, D. (1996). Quality and professionalism in health care: a review of current initiatives in the NHS. *British Medical Journal*, 312, 626–629.

Tripp, D. (1993). *Critical Incidents in Teaching: Developing Professional Judgement.* Routledge.

Chapter 4

Understanding artistry: educational research, practical enquiry and case study

Introduction

So far in this section we have shown that practice is inevitably 'messy', that it lies in what Schön (1987) calls 'the swampy lowlands' rather than residing at the heights of academe. We have demonstrated how we believe professionals to have been misled (by their education and by outsiders) to see their practice in technical terms and to believe that it can be brought under rational control, that its messiness can be cleared up if only professionals were better at their job, or if bureaucrats could bring professionals under greater (and stricter) regulation. We have pointed out that in current times matters are even worse. Now professionals like our contributors to this book carry the burden of believing that the only way to improve health care is for them to be involved in complex accountability and quality control procedures, because they have been told that professionals must account for what they do, and through this be *made* to improve. And so opportunities for self-regulation are receding fast.

We have argued for our contrasting belief that professional practice will improve only when professionals recognise (and accept) the messiness of their practice, learn how to understand it and thus learn new ways of living with it. We would wish to place emphasis on professionals understanding their practice better by means of learning to articulate its complexities. This enterprise should, we believe, be at the heart of professional development.

It is true that there is related to health itself (and to Public Health in particular) a vast scientific research industry dedicated to the extension of propositional (factual) knowledge about disease and its cures (although much more of this than the public – and some practitioners – realise is less like reliable fact than temporary theory). This information properly and importantly provides practitioners with new knowledge to apply in practice. That is, it contributes new knowledge for the practitioner to work with and in that way adds to the improvement of practice. But, our basic argument is, it does not help practitioners to refine their own practice.

We have shown that a professional's practice is informed more by his or her own personal practical knowledge than by formal knowledge which is external to the practitioner. Such personal knowledge is certainly very difficult to articulate – so difficult in fact that we tend to say that our practice 'comes with experience' and then leave it at that. We believe that there is great power in this knowledge in that it can inform our practice, and enable us to practise more effectively (though not necessarily more 'efficiently', which is about getting more for less and is often self-defeating). It also helps us to explain to our patients and clients, and to managers and politicians, our professional actions, and what has led to them. This is a different form of accountability from the technical one and it is arguably a wider version.

But how will understanding and being able to articulate one's practice improve it? Certainly not immediately, nor necessarily directly. There will be no short-term impact on practice (although there will be some on the practitioner). Deeper understanding of practice is not always demonstrable (let alone measurable), nor will improved practice necessarily or immediately cash out in terms of improved health outcomes. This is not about quick fixes but about longer term and more lasting benefits gained from the transformation of the professional whose development is based on greater awareness of what is involved in practice.

All this raises questions about how, in this view of professionalism, to be accountable and how to enquire into practice in ways that give due regard to its artistic nature and especially to the nature and significance of personal theory. This chapter will attempt to respond to these and show that by rigorous investigation of their practice which is recorded in forms that can be shared in public, practitioners can at the same time both fulfil the requirements of accountability, and lay a much sounder foundation for the improvement of their practice and their professional development than can ever be provided by bureaucratic regulation from outside. Such investigations are essentially educational. But they do not, as do the research approaches we discussed in Chapter 2, involve the extensive chasing and subsequent manipulation of empirical data (although this does not mean that such investigations are divorced from practice) nor do they demand the kind of extensive library searching that provides references for the sake of fulfilling academic course criteria (though they are not uninformed by formal theory). This means that they can be carried out by practitioners alongside their work and do not require major resources (apart from the time professionals find they are able to give it when they – and their managers – see it as a priority).

In short we argue for, and explain the procedures of, a form of enquiry beginning to be known as 'insider practitioner research', which is essentially educational, whose concern is with practical enquiry, and in which we take case study to be the most useful approach. This chapter will also act as an introduction to Part Two, in which the work of six professionals from a range of health care professions offers examples of this approach. We shall look firstly at accountability, secondly at new ways of seeing enquiry, thirdly at case study research as a key approach to insider practitioner research, and finally at the guidance we offered our colleagues. This will provide a context for reading their work in Part Two. (The means of rendering an *artistic* account of their work, together with the methods they drew upon to present and appreciate that account, emerge in Parts Two and Three and make better sense in that context. Their complexities are explored in detail in Fish, in press.)

Accountability

Currently health professionals (like many others) face the issue of accountability. This refers partly to the costs of health care, which universally are soaring. As advances in health care increase, the care that can be offered far outstrips the resources even in rich nations to provide for all those who might receive it. At the same time, there are calls for establishing measurable outcomes to health care. This approach ignores (deliberately or otherwise) the fact that much health care practice has tangible but immeasurable consequences, or even that the outcome of today's practice might not be observable for some time to come.

Professionals, then, are being called upon to justify their actions. They must keep up to date, they must incorporate best practice into their own work, they must become evidence-based. They must be accountable.

Yet the term accountability has two meanings. In the first sense it means that health professionals are expected **to account** *for* their actions. They must be held to account, to be judged for what they do. This approach to accountability is regulatory. It is a means for controlling professionals and their practice. Someone is checking up on what professionals do.

But there is a second version of accountability for health professionals, which fits a more self-regulatory view of professionalism. It also accords with what we have been arguing for in terms of professionals putting their actions into words, of explaining them, of helping themselves and others to understand better the nature of their practice. Here professionals voluntarily **give an account** *of* their practice. Such an account would, of course, need to go well beyond the factual and empirical level of the kind of account rendered (required) in audit and IPR. This will precisely enable the complexities of practice to be given proper weight and enable professionals to have their thoughts, ideas, paradoxes and dilemmas recognised.

In this book we take the second of these two meanings of the term accountability. At a time when professionals are being held to account for their actions, we will attempt to show what it means to ask professionals to understand and explain their practice through giving an account of what they do and why they do it. And we demonstrate how professionals can attempt to give such an account, by seeing their professionalism anew – as artistry, and the professional judgements they make as central to this. But what is the nature of this enterprise? And what principles and processes are involved in it?

The nature of the enterprise

Where the goal is improving understanding – whether practical or theoretical understanding – the enterprise is essentially educational even when the area in which improvement is to take place is in a profession well outside the teaching profession. That is, the intention to understand something implies the need to learn. This does not of course inevitably imply the need for a live teacher. There are many ways of coming to understand. And any teacher involved knows that it is not possible to 'give' someone understanding. This is something that each must work out for him or her self. But it does indicate that in seeking to extend understanding it is relevant to draw upon educational processes.

The significance of this is twofold. Firstly it makes it entirely appropriate that the approaches, methods and means utilised to extend understanding are drawn from, and that practitioners see themselves as working within, the broad traditions of *educational* research. Secondly because such enquiry will feed into accountability, research publications and professional development, it ensures that these are given an *educational* focus. That is, it will begin an important shift from seeing accountability, research and professional development as *administrative* chores to recognising their educational potential.

If this is the broad nature of the type of enquiry we are arguing for and offering examples of, what are the broad principles and procedures involved in it?

Some broad principles and processes involved

Trying to understand practice better is difficult, uncomfortable, takes time and is better worked on in respect of one small piece of practice rather than attempting a large-scale exploration. Yet in starting with a small but well chosen piece of his or her own practice a professional can quickly unravel some of the issues at its core and come to see them as relating to the heart of the profession's practice. The starting point for such enquiry, then, is intimate and highly detailed but it relates to wider issues and is ultimately for a public audience. This also helps practitioners to distance the account as it is worked over. And it does involve considerable re-working. Such re-working, we discovered in carrying through this project, needed particular support from us in respect of how to theorise practice and how to harness artistry of expression. We offered colleagues workshops on both of these. Fish (in press) provides further details of both processes. The whole enterprise is also helped – or at least supported – by working with a colleague or colleagues in a relationship known as 'critical friendship'. This consists of using the services of a colleague to act as a thoughtful (critical) audience to help check out and expand one's ideas and the theorising of one's practice as well as their presentation and communication in writing.

But there are no simple rules. Serious reflection on practice does not replace one dogma with another. It is something that one learns to do as one proceeds. Such research is itself an artistic process where neither the ends nor *the* specific means can be pre-specified. It is, rather, the principles which are important. Yet in spite of these demands, as is evident in the final part of this book, colleagues found the process liberating, exciting, helpful at a number of levels. Indeed, we know of no other activity in professional practice – apart from the rewards of practice itself – which at the same time fulfils the demands for accountability, research, and professional development and provides refreshment of mind and spirit.

But it is also hard (as is often the case with something rewarding). It is hard because it involves both looking at difficult matters and finding words that express them adequately. It involves revealing the depth of thought and feeling beneath our actions, because there is much that is ineffable, unspoken, unacknowledged during practice which needs to be articulated if it is ever to be learnt from and worked upon. It is for these reasons that we emphasise the help provided by both *seeing the artistry* in our practice and in *presenting with artistry* the story of that practice. We hope to show that by appreciating such art and by using artistry to share it with others, the understandings that arise can extend and provoke further debate, reshape public understanding and have impact upon the practitioner in profound ways.

This involves the need to argue with ourselves and deliberate (with others) – to engage in practical reasoning – about the dilemmas, the inevitably contestable issues that are endemic to professional practice. 'It involves improving practice through systematic critical enquiry where the term critical implies review leading to better understanding of practice and offering potential emancipation from existing traditions or established patterns of practice' (see Golby and Appleby, 1995).

By sharing these in public, professionals could ultimately reshape the public's perceptions of practice. And it can change practitioners too, since it increases awareness of the bases of professional actions, decisions, judgements. Primarily it enables professionals to see their practice anew, to recognise and articulate its complexities and the contestable notions and values that lie at its heart, and thus to learn to refine those things which can be developed and live with those which cannot. In other words, we believe that reflective practice focused upon appreciating the artistry of professional work can profoundly alter practitioners' understanding of practice and theory, equip them to be articulate about this, to think critically about it, to establish different priorities as the basis for practice, and thus effect far-reaching and well-founded changes to practice. We would hope that it might lead practitioners to challenge the notion of *evidence*-based practice and work towards the establishment of praxis (*morally*-based practice), and thus reinstate professionalism on a proper foundation.

Being articulate about the complexities of practice might, in a liberal view of accountability, satisfy the need to 'give an account', but could it ever count as research? How can it be seen as proper research or enquiry when it is neither scientific, nor large scale? How can it even be humanistic enquiry when there is little emphasis on data-gathering, less emphasis than usual (or certainly a different emphasis) on formal theory and when there are no straightforward conclusions for other practitioners to apply? And what, then, is the role of the audience for such 'research'? The following is an attempt to respond to these questions, to clarify the broad research traditions in order to show where such investigation of practice is located, and to indicate why the results of such a study should be of interest to other practitioners within health care and beyond (rather than merely to quality control administrators).

Research: clarifying the broad traditions

The general view about what counts as research held by many health care practitioners is as we have indicated in Chapter 2. Here the scientific paradigm is assumed automatically to be the starting point, even the epitome, of real research, and everything else is defined by contrast to that. This idea has also been handed down into educational research, so that even those who argue for survey, illuminative or action research often feel a need to do so by first expounding the case for and against scientific research.

But to anyone who knows about the history of ideas this is very ironic indeed. In fact it is only very recently in the history of ideas – only since the mid-nineteenth century – that the term 'theory' has come to be seen almost exclusively as scientific theory. Such scientific theory (often assumed to be absolute knowledge, and referred to usually as 'scientific knowledge') is the result of Scientific Research, which, by using empirical methods on a large scale makes discoveries, which are held at the time to be unassailable evidence, and which in turn are 'handed down' to practitioners to be put into operation in their practice until newer and apparently better knowledge is similarly discovered and handed down. As practitioners know well, this enterprise has produced a huge literature not only containing the results of this form of enquiry but also expounding on the processes and traditions, the values, beliefs and assumptions involved in this tradition of enquiry. For many – even for the recent research assessment exercise in universities – this is the only meaning of the term 'research', and (despite endless new discoveries which outdate previous ones) it is believed, or at least people behave as if it is believed, that such scientific research leads directly to new and permanent scientific knowledge. All other forms of theory, if they are recognised at all are considered of lesser value, and any other versions of enquiry are often not accorded the term 'research'.

But for thousands of years prior to this, knowledge was understood differently, and in fact it still is by those who penetrate beneath the surface of these issues. As Aristotle shows, that which we call 'Research' and think of as a scientific, empirical and action-based activity leads to a form of *theory* (usually theories about new ideas to apply to practice). In fact, although its means are highly active, being empirical, this 'scientific' research is called by Aristotle 'theoretical enquiry' in recognition of its goal of supplying new theory to practice.

But this 'theoretical enquiry' is only one form of enquiry. Different kinds of enquiry lead to different ends. Those means of enquiry which lead to an improved understanding of practice, and which are usually taken by practitioners themselves, Aristotle called 'practical enquiry'. This is concerned with promoting critical thinking about, and reflection on, practice. Such enquiry involves moral and practical reasoning and does not at all *rest* upon empirical enquiry, since moral decisions can never rest simply on empirical matters. This 'practical enquiry' concerns itself with consideration of the moral and ethical bases of action and takes account of the social, historical and political context of the action and the traditions of the broader practice in which that action is embedded. It is, thus, also values-related.

In other words, practical enquiry – improved understanding of practice – starts with practice and through this discovers theory and returns again to practice. It depends on practical reasoning and seeks to see holistically the particular activity of a practitioner within the broader tradition of which it is part. In doing so it has to recognise the problematic and contestable nature of the ideas upon which professional practice rests, and to admit that judgements about the decisions and about the activities of practice depend upon values – they are never quite simply right or wrong. Thus, ironically, although the ends of 'practical enquiry' are indeed practical, the means by which it achieves these are *less 'active'* and more cerebral than those of 'scientific' research which starts with theory, through it turns to practice and then returns to theory (that is, whose ends are theoretical and whose means are empirical). This 'practical enquiry' involves engaging those who are involved in enquiry into their *own* practice in a wider practical discourse, the processes of which are calculated to open up greater under-standing rather than designed to discover new knowledge, and the results of practical enquiry are not in the *application* to practice of *other peoples'* ideas but the refinement and development of one's own.

Thus, the audience for such research is at least as much self (the individual practitioner involved in enquiry) as it is others (other practitioners who will learn from it). And what each of these will learn is not new knowledge to apply to their practice but rather how to understand better their own practice. And this involves practitioners in two kinds of responsibilities: to take up, at the level of deliberation, the issues raised by such enquiry, and to reflect in a serious way upon (enquire into) their own practice. In this latter endeavour, the reflections of others (as provided in Part Two) offer an example of the kind of investigations that readers themselves might undertake. What they avowedly do not do is offer 'new knowledge' or even expert knowledge about the issues raised which readers can (let alone should) then apply to their own practice. And this also usefully and refreshingly frees insider practitioner researchers from being inhibited by the need to be an 'expert' on the issues they are grappling with. Indeed, as our contributors discovered, the only thing they can claim to be experts on is their own understanding of their own practice – and this understanding (and hence their expertise) is changing all the time.

Thus 'theoretical enquiry' and 'practical enquiry' are two separate enterprises, each offering something quite different, but of equal value to the professional practitioner, and each able to be harnessed to focus upon practice, but with different goals in mind. For this reason, the term 'practitioner researcher' is not alone sufficient to distinguish between them, and we have therefore adopted the rather awkward term currently prevalent, that of 'insider practitioner researcher' to denote the idea of the practitioner exploring the principles and processes of his or her own practice with a view to understanding it better. We are *not* saying that scientific theory (provided it is seen as 'theory' and not as absolute knowledge) is not vital for professionals. Clearly it is. And we are not saying that formal theory is unimportant for professional practice. Clearly it is too. We are saying that in addition to this, professionals need the activities of and the results of 'practical enquiry'. And those seeking to understand their own practice are therefore working within a perfectly honourable and long-standing tradition – that of practical enquiry. Table 4.1 provides a summary of these points.

If this is the broad tradition of research in which we work, what approaches best enable us to undertake such enquiry, what are the details of how to conduct such a study, and what broad processes did the authors of the following six chapters go through? We shall respond to the first two of these questions by reference to the very useful work of Golby (1993) – which again we cannot do full justice to here, and the full version of which we commend to our readers. Finally we shall provide very brief details of the very limited guidance that we offered to our colleagues. We shall then leave our readers to gain a much richer sense of what is involved by reading our colleagues' work in Part Two. And in Part Four, Chapter 14, we shall tease out from the experience of our colleagues some ideas which seemed useful to them after they had been through the process.

Table 4.1   Practical enquiry and theoretical enquiry

Characteristics	Theoretical enquiry	Pratical enquiry
Values	Truth/explanation of facts	The good of patients, clients/learners
Goals	Knowledge	Understanding
Focus	Discovering new propositional knowledge	Uncovering the moral and ethical bases of own actions and professional practice
View of theory/practice	Disengaged from practioners' practice	Sees practice as of prime importance
Status of researcher	Expert in knowledge generation	Practioner is not expert on issues. Knows about and learns more about learning in own practice
Function of academe	To train/coach researchers. To be the repository and disseminators of propositional knowledge	To enhance the knowledge-creating capacity of practitioners
Nature of enquiry	Scientific – to generate unassailable evidence. Action-based action leading to theory (ideas)	Moral enquiry, critical thinking and reflection to aid in understanding. This leads to refined practice
Processes	Empirical enquiry – uses large scale research methods to discover 'unassailable' empirical evidence	Small scale and not only empirical but moral reasoning – deliberates about issues – uncovers uncertainty
Leading to	Speculative theorising, also applying theory to others' practice	Practical discourse, and practical action
Audience and their responsibilities	Practioners as 'others', application of others' theory to their practice	Practitioners (self and others) to engage in moral enquiry about others' issues and own practice

Case study: a basis for practical enquiry

In considering the three most obvious approaches to research that were readily available to practitioners who wished to understand their practice and who saw their practice as akin to artistry, we saw illuminative enquiry, action research and case study as possibilities. Both illuminative enquiry and action research are founded firmly in the humanistic paradigm in which the social sciences provide the main methods and tools. We concluded though that case study makes better provision for focusing on practical enquiry, and particularly that it better respected the artistry of practice. It is aimed at understanding practice in all its complexity and sees practice as part of the history and as shaped by the traditions of the practice of a profession. Case study thus places emphasis upon reflection and deliberation, on context and meaning. By comparison, illuminative enquiry focuses on the social world of practice, placing emphasis on data collection in community settings and being interested in illuminating these, and action research seeks from the outset to change practice and places emphasis on present data and theories of change, thus being more interested in a radical intervention than in understanding the present and its traditions and the potential for change from within. We therefore consider case study research as particularly appropriate to this work and we asked the contributors to make this the basis of the work presented in Part Two, sharing with them Golby's arguments.

Golby argues persuasively that, 'properly conceived, [case study] is uniquely appropriate as a form of educational research for practitioners to conduct', having the potential 'to relate theory and practice' and 'advancing professional knowledge' by academically respectable means (Golby, 1993, p. 3). But, he warns, 'case study is too often misconceived', and it is therefore important to understand the rationale for it.

Golby, quoting the work of Yin, argues that case study involves practice rather than philosophical enquiry. He draws from this three important points. These are that case study is an approach to research and not a method, that within this approach it is 'an open question what methods are to be used', and that it is not necessarily only qualitative methods that are acceptable. He argues rather that 'methods should be dictated by the need to understand, not selected on doctrinal grounds' (Golby, 1993, p. 5). In this sense, he is arguing that case study cuts across the normal research paradigms. This allows us to argue that to understand the ineffable, complex, messy and human and to some extent mysterious aspects of professional practice – those aspects in which the artistry of the professional is emphasised and within which judgement is a central feature – it is appropriate to use artistic methods within the case study approach. It also spares us arguing here the case for using such methods which are drawn from a world of research that is not (as yet) enshrined in a research paradigm recognised in practitioner research, and which therefore merit a lengthy explanation. (See Fish, in press, for an elaboration of these issues.) Instead we shall, in accordance with our belief in the primacy of practice, leave our colleagues' work to demonstrate the principles and processes involved.

Golby also argues that 'case study is appropriate where it is not yet clear what are the right questions to ask'. And in these terms too, case study seems an appropriate approach for the kind of insider practitioner research with a practical enquiry thrust that we have in mind. This is because it involves a practitioner exploring in depth his or her own practice in such a way that it is very likely that the really important questions endemic to it will arise only at the end of the study. He adds:

> There needs to be a sense of perplexity, problems to be addressed, and a sense of the researcher's interest in these problems. But premature closure is inimical to good case study. (Golby, 1993, p. 5)

He adds a little later:

> it will start from some provisional understanding of the case and investigate it further. (p. 5)

Golby also argues that 'a case must be an example of something'. The cases presented in Part Two below are all cases of practitioners articulating and exploring a small part of their practice (which itself is characterised by artistry) and where a problem or issue 'brought them up short', or in Schön's term caused them some 'surprise', in such a way that they could identify an incident that crystallised the larger complexities of their work. By articulating in detail the incident they were enabled to see that problem in relation to a wider set of ideas – both within their own individual professional practice and in the traditions of the practice of their profession. Such an incident, then, provided for them a particular example of a more generalisable issue, problem or dilemma.

Golby notes the importance of seeing case study as the study of *particularity* rather than of uniqueness. He declares that claiming that case study is about portraying uniqueness is a serious error. In understanding a case it is necessary to see it in, and relate it in some way to, a wider context. It is only because it is possible to see it as an example of a general case that it is possible to say anything at all about it. If a case or incident within it were *unique*, such that nothing like it had ever been seen, it would be impossible to see to what it related, and thus impossible to make sense of it, beyond staring at it in wonder. Golby quotes Elton: 'the unique event is a freak or a frustration' (Golby, 1993, pp. 7–8). If, by contrast, the case is seen as a particular manifestation of a general case, then both its individual nature and its generic nature can be discussed.

It is in this articulating of particular examples of practice that we believe there is a need for a conscious drawing upon artistic methods and styles, since the case being investigated is, by definition, an example of professional artistry. But such an enquiry would, of course, include inspecting the basis of this judgement too. We need to ask as part of such investigations: is professional practice inherently artistic? We need, too, to be aware of the basis of our own values, beliefs and assumptions even as we frame these issues. Golby notes: 'You must believe something at the outset, in order that you believe more and quite different things as you proceed' (Golby, 1993, p. 9).

Part of this also involves a need to be aware of the context (historical, professional, political, cultural, social) and thus to be able to 'place' the case in wider traditions. And it is here, in relating the case to the wider issues and understandings, and *not* in excavating and articulating the particular, that the perspectives of formal theory make their real contribution. It is not, as Golby says, 'having a body of knowledge that is the hallmark of professional activity, but the accessing of that knowledge in relation to particular cases' (Golby, 1993, p. 11). So research of this kind entails moving from the particular case to general knowledge and understanding and back again in a continual iteration.

Descriptive, interpretative and critical case study

It is an axiom of art that form and content work in unison towards the same end, and that the structure of the work is therefore one way into beginning to understand its intentions. So, too, the basic shape or composition of a case study will convey its nature. A case study which offers substantial details of the case but little more, is likely to be a **descriptive case study**, offering one interpretation of the experience. By contrast, a study in which the detail is set in a wider context, and where the local description (at all its levels) yields at various points to an interpretation of a case, to various differing perspectives on it, is **reflective (or interpretative) case study**. Both of these are in contrast to the **deliberative (or critical) case study** where the writer's priorities are the deliberations and emerging critical perspectives which arise from the narrative. It is, of course, the latter two kinds (interpretative and critical case studies) which are offered by our contributors in Part Two. The role of theorising practice and of formal theory in each different case will be obvious to any reader who looks out for these aspects. But the distinctions between reflection and deliberation perhaps need further clarification.

Reflection and deliberation

Our preferred definition of reflection is that which is endemic to the term reflective practice. This involves a careful consideration of one's own practice by means of systematic critical enquiry. It aims at better understanding of practice, involves standing back from it and offers the possibility of dissociation from existing traditions or established patterns of practice (see above p. 59 and also Golby and Appleby, 1995). This is about reviewing (re-viewing) practice in all its aspects. Essentially reflection concerns thinking about actions and thoughts relating to action. Schön, whose writings on reflection are seminal, tries to distinguish between reflection-in and reflection-on action. He defines the former as 'questioning the assumptional structure of knowing-in-action' ... as thinking critically about 'the thinking that got us into this fix or this opportunity' (Schön, 1987, p. 28). Boud, Keogh and Walker indicate that such processes can be useful in the preparation, during engagement in an activity, and in the processing of what has been experienced' (Boud *et al.*, 1985, p. 9).

By comparison, deliberation is another term for practical reasoning, and goes beyond the critical consideration of one's practice itself and one's thinking during it, to focus on the problematic and contestable *issues* endemic to practising as a professional. Here, Schwab, whose work is seminal, offers the following:

> Deliberation is complex and arduous. It treats both ends and means and must treat them as mutually determining one another. It must try to identify, with respect to both, what facts may be relevant.

He adds:

> Deliberation requires consideration of the widest possible alternatives if it is to be most effective. (Schwab, 1970, pp. 318–319)

Here then we see that deliberation concerns itself with moral and ethical issues, with ends as well as means, and thus emphasises a key dimension in the investigation of practice which reflection alone does not emphasise.

It is by working on (reflecting about and deliberating on) the presentation of their descriptions of practice by challenging beliefs, customs and rituals, and then by investigating the issues that arise, that health care practitioners can understand and thence refine their practice. Indeed, in theorising their practice they are opening it and their concomitant theorising to public scrutiny. As Kemmis reminds us:

> Practices are judged by publicly shared criteria and traditions, by reference to the lives, virtues and excellencies of practitioners as the bearers of these traditions, and by reference to the works of institutions created to nurture and sustain these activities and values, virtues and excellencies they embody and express. (Kemmis, 1995, p. 15)

The case studies in Part Two

It is time now to provide the final details which will enable readers to respond to and judge the contributions of our colleagues and through them the veracity of our claims about this kind of research. (But this, we would remind you, is only a preliminary to the more important matters of you the reader taking up the issues in deliberation with colleagues and of reflecting upon your own practice.) We thus offer, finally, the details with which our writers set out on their adventure of writing about their practice.

The practitioners with whom we were privileged to work on this project volunteered or were invited from amongst professionals with whom we had already worked in professional development and who shared our frustration that there were no examples in health care of published case studies of the kind we describe. Basically we worked with them over a period of fifteen months during which we met on eight occasions, sometimes for discussions, sometimes for rather more formal workshops which we offered in response to their early drafts, or, as in the case of the final one, where we shared with them and gained their responses to our contributions to the book. At the beginning, as we began to word the proposal to the publisher, we offered our colleagues some guide-lines and then worked away from these, and far beyond them, making new meanings together as we went. During those occasions and in intermediate meetings we, as editors, worked out, shared and clarified the ideas which we have outlined in these opening chapters of this book. And we offered some further details to our colleagues on theorising practice and about artistry (as indicated above and in Fish, in press).

The ideas we began with were tentative and the three main pieces of information we offered them, developed by Della, were never intended to be more than the broadest of guidance for working on case studies. We offered details of how to identify so called 'critical incidents' with which we asked them to begin their writing (see below, Box 4.1 and Box 4.2) and some simple suggestions on developing a case study (Box 4.3). We include these three boxes at the end of this chapter in case readers prefer to look first at the case studies themselves before returning to the frameworks that we ten-tatively offered our colleagues.

The flavour of what our contributors made to the discussions and the mutual support they gave each other is clearly identified and can be easily recognised in the work which follows. And it is now time that we allowed it to speak for itself.

References

Boud, D., Keogh, R. and Walker, D. (eds.) (1985). *Reflection: Turning Experience into Learning*. Kogan Page.

Fish, D. *Appreciating Practice in the Caring Professions: Re-focusing Professional Development and Practitioner Research*. Butterworth–Heine-mann. In press.

Golby, M. (1993). *Case Study as Educational Research*. Fair Way Publications.

Golby, M. and Appleby, R. (1995). Reflective practice through critical friendship: some possibilities. *Cambridge Journal of Education*, 25, 149–160.

Kemmis, S. (1995). Prologue: theorising educational practice. In *For Education: Towards Critical Educational Enquiry* (W. Carr, ed.), pp. 1–17. Open University Press.

Schön, D. (1987). *Educating the Reflective Practitioner*. Jossey-Bass.

Schwab, J. J. (1970). The practical: a language for curriculum. In *Science, Curriculum, and Liberal Education: Selected Essays* (I. Westbury and N. J. Wilkof, eds.), pp. 287–321. University of Chicago Press.

Box 4.1   Critical incidents: an overview

What is a critical incident?

Critical incidents were originally used by historians.

A critical incident is an event whose significance has been produced by the way we look at it.

Focusing upon and reflecting upon an event in one's professional practice can aid the development of professional judgement.

It is a useful starting point for refining the focus of a project or enquiry.

Using critical incidents is about learning to see and to be more aware of aspects of our practice – *and* of the limitations of how we see practice.

It is about learning to see our practice in a new light. This involves:

- investing some significance in an event via the way we see it (that is, via the way we *interpret* it, since all seeing is value-laden and blinkered by what we bring to it)
- and then probing the theories through which we see it and trying to see it and them in new ways;
- recognising the problematic nature of it and of practice generally.

A critical incident can be a highly significant event with important consequences or – more likely – a commonplace event that occurs during routine practice.

A critical incident can be drawn from:

- a routine piece of practice (that which we have mainly stopped noticing);
- an event which we have noticed in passing during practice because it was: funny; sad; interesting; amusing; boring; silly; witty; violent; surprising; annoying; pleasing; typical; atypical.

It will be rendered critical by the means of analysis/interpretation/appreciation, which sees it as an example of a category in a wider – usually social – context.

Box 4.1 (*continued*)

Its significance will be that it is indicative of underlying trends /theories/beliefs/assumptions – perhaps that it is *typical* rather than 'critical'.

This whole process also confronts us with our habits and with the inevitably contradictory notions and aspects of our own practice and our ideas about it.

It also provides a means of setting a new practical agenda.

Box 4.2   Critical incidents: some useful questions

First, pin-point and then describe an incident as vividly as possible.

Provide a narrative in chronological order of the events and processes of the practical situation (what happened, and what you felt, thought and did about it).

NB: It should be noted that recapturing or reconstructing a complex situation chronologically in this way is not always easy, or straightforward. The mind/memory does not work like this. However, a disciplined attempt to relive/reconstruct an incident, preferably soon after the event, will usually enable it to be ordered into a narrative. Such a process often enables the learner-practitioner to recognise for the first time what actually has happened. It also establishes a basis from which further reflection can grow.

Then analyse and interpret it. Here the following questions might help.

Ask what else might have happened – or what else *should* have happened?
Try to see it from another viewpoint.
Ask what didn't happen.
Consider what really was the cause of the problem.
Consider a reversal of the situation.
Consider what has been left out of the story you have told.
Ask what personal theories (espoused theories and theories-

Box 4.2 (*continued*)

in-use), and what beliefs, values and assumptions lie under the incident.

Finally, consider carefully:

What are the problematic notions involved here, what are the dilemmas being posed by the incident, what is it that is essentially contestable and unresolvable?

What needs further consideration? What is to be learnt from this?

Box 4.3   You *are* a real case! Practitioner research and its processes

Reflective practitioners (by some definitions) commit themselves to investigating their *own* practice with a view to understanding it better and to improving it. The following are the likely constituents of this process – neither temporal order nor hierarchical order should be read into the list below. They are *not* entirely discrete processes.

The homing-in process:

- identifying an issue or aspect of *personal* practice currently seen as important which needs working on and where such work would benefit that practice
- reflecting on aspect/issue with a view to identifying *why/for whom* it is important

Crystallising the issue/problem:

- capturing on paper – *briefly,* but as vividly as possible – a critical incident (one or more) which is/are *illustrative of and central to* the issue/problem – and considering critically both the incident, *and the values implicit in the writing*
- constructing a contextual analysis /clarifying the context in which the incident arose and considering critically both it *and the values implicit in the construction*

Box 4.3 (*continued*)

- further highlighting the issue/problem and thinking critically about how it *relates* to the critical incident(s)
- taking account of one's own personal beliefs, values, perspectives as part of the incident

Identifying the *nature* of the problem/issue

- examining and appreciating the nature of the problem (practical, prudential?)
- considering the nature of the issue and thus the *kinds of questions it generates*
- analysing and/or interpreting the problem/issue
- thinking critically about the issue/problem, the critical incident/ and the context

Investigating the matter further both theoretically and practically:

The order of these processes will be relevant to the topic being investigated, the possibilities for investigation and the values of the investigator.

- exploring theoretical perspectives
  - personal theory
  - relevant formal theory
  - overall parameters (ongoing literature search & review)

The order you choose here says things about your values.

- exploring own ongoing practice (decide methods/tools)
  - range of small-scale research techniques

Clarifying/interpreting/thinking critically

- making meaning out of the problem, its context, the investigations and the values
- planning for the future.

NB: This paper makes no suggestions about the structure, or any other aspect of your resulting written presentation

Part Two

Exploring Professional Judgement

Chapter 5

Taken for granted

Rosemary Richardson

Introduction

The particular incident to be described occurred during the summer of 1995 and concerns a personal experience with implications for my practice as a nurse teacher. The background to the incident will be described in order to 'set the scene' and the various factors which appeared to influence it will be explored. An attempt will be made to illustrate the complexities of such situations and my interpretation of what the implications appear to be, both for my own practice and for education and health care practice in more general terms. In order to avoid clumsy repetition, the term 'nurse' is used in place of 'nurse, midwife or health visitor'.

Most of my 'nursing practice' experience has been in non-institutional settings, mainly as a health visitor. A significant feature in relation to this incident is that my current teaching responsibilities include contributing to the community health studies components of diploma and degree level courses for pre- and post-registration student nurses. This includes liaison and negotiation ('networking') with a wide range of both professional and lay personnel involved in students' learning opportunities relating to community experience.

The critical incident

The background to the incident

My very elderly father, a retired priest and schoolmaster aged ninety-one years, had been admitted to the elderly care unit of a local community hospital five days previously. He had suffered from a chronic irritation of his skin for some time which had been treated by the general practitioner (GP). The condition had become worse over the past year, resulting in very disturbed nights whereby my mother, herself in her eighties, had become exhausted. She had previously declined offers of respite care, feeling that this would make my father feel abandoned and that, in any case, it was her responsibility to care for him. The accumulation of her exhaustion resulted in my father needing to be admitted the same day that my mother recognised the need for a break. She hoped that a cause could be found for the skin irritation. Despite regular visits, at least twice a day, no information had been offered to my mother since my father's admission. There were also other concerns about the standard of care, such as the hearing aid being incorrectly inserted or not inserted at all, spectacles being 'lost', fluids placed out of reach, inadequate clothing, despite warm clothing being available, heavily soiled clothing (not previously or subsequently such a frequent problem at home) left for my mother to take home and deal with before it could be washed. However, although these issues are not the subject of this particular incident I was (and still am) left wondering what action, if any, I should or should not have taken and am conscious of the tensions between my professional responsibilities and my personal obligations not to create possible friction in what is quite a small community and where my mother continues to live. I am also aware of the impact the experience has had on my practice as a teacher which is why the incident has been chosen for exploration.

A meeting

I lived some three hours' car drive from my parents and went to stay with my mother for the weekend following my father's admission to hospital. Because of our increasing frustration about the lack of information, my mother agreed that I should make an appointment for us to see the doctor responsible for the unit, on the Monday morning, the fifth day following admission. This involved my unexpectedly having to take a further 'special carers' leave' day off work. I was fortunate to have an employer and colleagues who consistently provided genuine support throughout the lengthy period of time that various incidents, including the one being discussed, occurred. However, there is a potential dilemma for both employers and employees, in caring organisations, in terms of the dual roles in which employees can find themselves.

During the discussion with the doctor, he assured us that there was 'really nothing medically wrong' with my father other than old age, but that 'they' could certainly improve his mobility by at least 15 per cent.

It was at that moment that I realised that there were two very different agendas. Ours was the one discussed earlier. 'The professionals' clearly saw the problem as one of mobility. When my mother mentioned the skin irritation, she was informed that, yes, 'they' were aware of it but were not sure of the cause. My father had therefore been treated for a possible parasitic skin condition and the results of the skin tests were expected back 'within a few days'. The comments then reverted to my father's mobility 'problems'. I asked my mother, during the meeting, if she had been involved in any discussions during my father's admission. She said that she had not been consulted by either doctors or nurses, other than to confirm the name and address on the admission documents.

We had been assured by the doctor that the GP and the district nurses had been concerned about my father's mobility. This might have been the case with the GP who had arranged my father's admission since he was not my father's own GP. However, I knew that the district nurses were well aware of the situation which made me wonder if they had either not been involved adequately or perhaps their views had not been 'heard'.

On our return to the ward, I asked if we could meet the primary nurse but was told that team nursing was the approach in use. The full stop was literal. I then asked to see the named nurse. Some time later, a nurse arrived. There was no introduction, merely a rather surprised statement that, "You wanted to see me, did you?" The nurse listened politely to my mother but there was no sense that her dedicated care of my father in very difficult circumstances was respected nor that her 'expert' knowledge about my father's condition and needs was valued or relevant. Similarly, it did not appear to be recognised that she might, as a carer, have needs of her own and was not just the collector of soiled clothes hanging on the end of the bed in a plastic bag.

Prior to his admission, my father had for some time needed a considerable amount of help with dressing and undressing and with his personal hygiene. He had had an indwelling catheter inserted for about two months. This he disliked but most of the time he tolerated it with an air of resigned acceptance. Despite the hospital doctor's critical opinion about the catheter, its use had helped to restore some of the dignity which, often severe, urge incontinence had undermined. It had also reduced the pressures on my mother in terms of time spent helping my father to change and washing his clothes. Although my father's mobility was limited he had still been managing to walk slowly round the ground floor of the house and to go upstairs to bed. He had worn glasses for many years and his hearing was partially impaired. He was confused at times but he was also very aware of his increasing frailty which he found frustrating and depressing, often expressing the wish that, 'the Good Lord' would take him. All of these issues could have emerged through a thorough assessment.

Immediate reactions

As we left the hospital, I felt a mixture of dismay, disbelief and consternation. A key element relating to my teaching concerns the encouragement of holistic and individualised assessments encompassing a partnership approach during which the contributions of the client and the professional are of equal value. This includes encouraging students to listen and to take account of a patient or client's personal, family and community circumstances and the factors which influence them. My role includes working as a member of a team to provide a range of practical and academic learning opportunities. This includes discussion of experiences, reference to research and other publications, and assignments. Indeed, the purpose of a recently introduced Study of Health in the Community assignment for pre-registration students is, 'for students to develop awareness of the importance of valuing patients and clients as individuals and as members of families and communities and to recognise the implications ... for their nursing practice'.

Evaluations of the learning experiences in the community suggest that students gain much, both personally and professionally, from these opportunities and recognise the implications for practice.

What *was* happening in the reality of 'hospital' practice? I had read of the excellent work reportedly occurring in a number of areas, based on humanistic and holistic principles, for example at Burford Community Hospital (Pearson, 1991). Surely these examples were not exceptions? Where were we going wrong? Were all my ideals in vain?

It is, however, a different matter to write chronologically about an incident in retrospect when, at the time, one's thoughts resemble the lottery numbers tumbling about, before they drop into line, still out of order, waiting to be put in the 'right order'. As we walked through the car park, my head was full of thoughts about Thomas's (1976) words concerning how situations are defined, of Blumer's reference to the 'gravest kind of error' arising from substituting our own meanings (Blumer, 1969, p. 51), of the confusion and misunderstandings which arise when the 'two parties' do not understand each other (Blumer, 1969, p. 9). This thinking was influenced by my studies during my M.Ed. course in Exeter. Phrases which made an impact whilst reading the work of writers to whom I was 'introduced' often come into my mind when I find myself in challenging situations. Prior to the course (and since), I have often felt it had been implied by my family and colleagues that my thinking was rather non-conformist in relation to theirs – at least, that was (and is) my interpretation. I felt, during the course, that I had at last 'found' a community of thinking which reflected my own beliefs and values but expressed them in ways to which I felt I could never aspire. The words referred to above came into my mind at the time of the incident when they were given an unforeseen and dramatic significance. It was apparently 'taken for granted' that mobility was the key problem but as Schutz suggests, 'a change of attention can transform something taken for granted into something problematical' (Schutz, 1972, p. 74). This phrase was therefore 'borrowed' for the title for this chapter, again because of its significance.

It was subsequently found that my father was very anaemic on account of a bone marrow condition and that his skin irritation was attributable to the complications caused by his illness. He died, at home, one month after the meeting at the hospital with the doctor and nurse.

What was only a brief incident has a wealth of personal and professional implications concerning both practice and theory. It provides the opportunity for exploring them through a process of reflective, critical enquiry which attempts to offer differing viewpoints and relate them to theories and other relevant literature which may 'shed light' on the circumstances and their interpretation. It does not involve using a reflective 'model' for reasons which I hope will become apparent.

Reflecting about the incident

Thinking, and writing, reflectively and critically analytically about experiences from our professional practice is something which has slowly been gaining support and credibility within a number of professions, for example, teaching and nursing. It also has its critics. Accusations of 'if we did that all the time we'd never get anything done', 'we do it anyway', 'it's being subjective' and comments such as 'students *must* learn to write using a proper academic style' have been levelled against it. To write about a *personal* experience might seem to be the ultimate academic crime.

The incident described above suggested to me that perhaps it was time we stopped trying to negate the influence of personal experiences in terms of our practice and confronted the issue 'up front'. The decision to take this step has been influenced by two particular experiences. These may be referred to as 'intellectual' and 'practical' but are closely linked and perhaps illustrate a need to challenge the conventional, technical rational, view of theory in nurse education as something to be applied (apparently uncritically) to practice, seeing it instead as something that is fundamentally integral with practice. As suggested by the guidance notes for a course assignment about reflective professional practice which I submitted as a student, 'theory is the understanding ("under-standing") of our practice' (Golby, 1992). Similarly, Oakeshott refers to theorising as 'an engagement of understanding' during which, he suggests, we search for evidence, explore connections and attempt to understand an occurrence as an 'intelligible event' (Oakeshott, 1975, p. 106).

Implicit in this suggestion is the relevance of personal theory. Fish and Purr, in their evaluation of practice-based learning in post-registration nurse education courses, found the definition of theory to be mostly narrow, that 'no one had heard of personal theory' and that few people recognised that 'theory can come from practice as well as being applied to it' (Fish and Purr, 1991, p. 66). This is not to detract, however, from the important influence of 'theory-in-the-literature' (Bassey, 1990), on our thinking and our practice. Some of the literature which has influenced me will now be discussed. It illustrates, for me, a community of thinking which is of particular relevance to the incident, and therefore to practice more widely. It is also part of my own attempt to explore connections and gain a greater understanding of the event.

The critical incident: immediate considerations

Influential experiences

One of my more important 'intellectual' experiences was gained through being introduced to the works of Schutz, whose work was much influenced by Husserl. He suggests that we define situations from the perspective of our own experiences, our own biography. He suggests that our position at any one time is not only related to our role and status within a social system (Schutz, 1970, p. 67) but also to our moral (ethical) and ideological position. Schutz (1967) also suggests that if we are looking at the experiences of another person, everything we 'know' about them is based on our own experiences. What are put forward as 'objective' views have begun subjectively but we then attempt to make them general. We hide ourselves behind an impersonal 'someone'. What has led to the views is considered to be no longer relevant.

This, of course, has considerable implications for professional practice. It is almost a daily occurrence to hear reference to the need for practitioners to be 'objective', thus reinforcing the need for this particular value to underpin professional practice; to be subjective is seen as unprofessional. As Williams suggests, 'a sense of something shameful, or at least weak, attaches to subjective' (Williams, 1976, p. 263), and, according to that view, subjective factors have to be 'put in their place' despite acceptance that they exist. The increasing value attached to reflective writing, albeit about professional experiences, represents a substantial movement in thinking, within the professions. The risk inherent in this form of writing, however, is when it becomes a technical search for elusive solutions to 'problems' rather than an increase in understanding of the complex issues involved.

The other experience to influence my choice of incident relates to research I undertook as part of a masters degree course. This concerned the role of personal tutor in nurse education. The evidence was gained through tape-recorded interviews with the various 'actors' concerned with the role. The transcripts of the interviews were analysed using a modified grounded theory approach. One of the findings, the significance of which I had not fully anticipated, came from the interviews with teachers who acted as personal tutors. When asked what had influenced them, in their role, each one of them referred to personal experiences of their own, as a student. For example, what one did now is 'based on what I've had in the past'. Another had had help and guidance in 'such a brilliant way' that 'when I was in the same position, I thought I would try to be the same'. Their comments suggested the significance of personal theory and its influence on practice.

The reasons for my choice of a personal experience as a critical incident therefore relate, in part, to the words of Schutz, amongst others, and in part to the findings from my research. Both examples suggest, to me, that we should not deny that particular personal experiences influence our practice but that we should acknowledge their influence, amongst a range of other varied experiences, recognising their contribution to increasing our understanding of the values and assumptions underpinning our practice and how it might be improved by the increased understanding.

The personal context

My father had been brought up in a clerical family which had a strong evangelical influence. He himself, however, was attracted by the more anglo-catholic traditions. As his obituaries stated, his philosophy was based on a deep sense of humanity, strong Christian principles and the ethic of hard work. As was also stated, he was not prepared to compromise these ideals, which could be linked to the early headmasters of Rugby and Uppingham Schools. They had promoted public and independent schools as 'Christian institutions and guardians of moral life' (Peterson, 1957, p. 55). These factors had a strong influence on his roles as a priest and as a schoolmaster. Mead, amongst others, stresses the need to consider the social contexts which give rise to the actions of individuals. As he suggests, 'the traces of past experience are continually playing in upon our perceived world' (Mead, 1962, p. 113). This is something I often recognise as happening in particular situations. The echoes can be almost audible.

I had been born at a public school and brought up in a cathedral choir school, both representing Peterson's views and what Dewey refers to as 'genuine community life' (Dewey, 1970 [1910], p. 16). However, Dewey expressed concern that an academic education results in future citizens with no sympathy for manual work and no understanding of 'the most serious of present day social and political difficulties' (Dewey and Dewey, 1915, p. 315). He was also concerned, for different reasons, about those who only had a 'trade training'. His concerns are of relevance to the incident described for a number of reasons.

The social context

Nursing was seen to be a suitable occupation for me, in terms of its vocational ideals and the appropriateness of its role orientation which, at that time, was implicit in the handmaiden image of nurses (mainly women) and of doctors (mainly men). Such influences have deeply rooted historical and cultural influences. One such example may be seen in the Biblical reference to the need for women to 'learn in silence with all subjection' and 'not to teach, nor to usurp authority over the man' (1 Timothy, 2.11,12) and, much later, Queen Victoria's fury at the 'mad, wicked folly of "Woman's Rights" .... God created men and women different – then let them remain each in their own position' (Queen Victoria, 1870). These views are in conflict with the values which I have come to hold, such as the need to avoid discriminating, for example, on grounds of gender or race, and for equality of opportunity and treatment regardless of circumstance. They also illustrate factors which have influenced, and continue to influence, how nursing is perceived by some professional and lay people, since nursing is still a predominantly female occupation.

Professional experiences

Despite such initial influences in my life, I began to find that my previous acceptance of the hierarchies and constraints of hospital life was no longer compatible with my developing beliefs and values. I subsequently worked in a variety of non-institutional settings, finally settling for a course leading to qualification as a health visitor. My practical experience during the course, and following it, occurred in West London where I was introduced to the second of Dewey and Dewey's descriptions. I came into contact with disadvantages and deprivations, and people of many nationalities and faiths, which would have been unimaginable had I remained within the shelter of my previous home and work environments. These experiences led me to question the basis of the values underpinning what I came to realise had been a narrow, cloistered existence. Not surprisingly, this sometimes resulted in situations where the two cultures came into conflict. I therefore find myself wondering about the extent to which these factors influence my approach to practice and the way I act within my present 'world'.

As a nurse teacher, whose professional experience has been predominantly community rather than hospital oriented, I am acutely aware of the gap that can sometimes occur between approaches to practice in each setting. As I write this, I find myself reflecting on the significance of the word 'acutely' and wonder if I should change it to one which sounds less emotive. It was written from the heart. Perhaps it would be better to write it from 'the head' – or not to write it at all. But 'acutely' summarises my feelings. Perhaps to ignore the significance of such a word may result in a 'papering over the cracks' in terms of trying to achieve greater understanding? Perhaps it offers a clue to my reaction to the incident described. Are there implications for how I see my role in trying to represent community interests in an institution which has its roots as a school for preparing students to work in hospital settings only? And what about the disagreements which arise with colleagues who do not share my values or perhaps see things from a different perspective? These can also give rise to feelings of 'acute' discomfort.

Some intellectual influences

The major significance which our experiences have for all of us, is suggested by Blumer. He explores and develops the concept of 'symbolic interactionism', whereby meaning comes through the process of interacting with others. However, he does not see meaning as having a psychological basis so much as a social basis and that social interaction is 'between *people* and not between roles' (Blumer, 1969, p. 75). Our understandings, or meanings, therefore, may be seen as a process of interpretation. This contrasts with the current culture in which interactions are so often interpreted in terms of behavioural performance. Blumer also warns against the supposedly 'objective' approach and goes on to suggest that it is necessary to find out how a person has 'defined the situation' in order to understand their actions. He further suggests that we risk setting up a 'fictitious world' if we substitute our own meanings instead of recognising the meanings held by the people concerned, in a particular situation. He goes so far as to refer to such substitution as 'the gravest kind of error that the social scientist can commit' (Blumer, 1969, p. 51). I recognise that I could be accused of just such an 'error', in terms of this discussion, since it is viewed only from my perspective rather than also exploring the perspective of the professionals involved. The practitioners involved with my father's assessment might have seen the approach used by them to be entirely appropriate. For the reasons described earlier, I have felt inhibited from raising the issue with them.

The meaning we give to an experience is not 'fixed'. It can vary depending on the circumstances at the time of the particular reflection. So what is the reality of a situation at any given time? I find it reassuring that Schutz himself admits that he, too, does not know and that he is comforted by knowing that he shared this 'unpleasant situation' with 'the greatest philosophers of all time' (Schutz, 1964, p. 88). However, this view is not shared by those who subscribe to a natural science perspective, whereby reality is seen as external to individuals and people are seen as puppets within efficient systems guided by rules which can be prescribed. This is in contrast to seeing people as capable of negotiating alternative meanings, able to act spontaneously, preferring to work 'with' rather than 'on' people (Fish, 1989). As I write that, I can find parallels between the former and the standards and audits which are currently being devised and implemented within a wide range of organisations including the health service. Similarly, the word 'competence' is frequently used in the assessment of nursing practice. What does it mean? As Hyland suggests, the notion of competence carries with it notions of '"lowest common denominator" characteristics' (Hyland, 1994, p. 19). Is that what we are willing to accept?

A harsh summary of my father's care could be seen in terms of him being given a bed in a modern, well-equipped ward, offered food at meal times and made the subject of some medical investigations, in effect treated as a puppet or, in Schutz's words as 'a conceptual model, not a real person' (Schutz, 1967, p. 242). Is this really the level of 'competence' we should seek to achieve? Is it illustrating a lack of understanding and familiarity with the reality of all the current pressures on practitioners, to have higher expectations? At a more complex level, was the impersonality of my father's treatment an example of the 'disembedding mechanism', the removal of social relations from local contexts referred to by Giddens, within an 'expert system' (the health service) which may be seen to be part of the nature of modernity? (See Giddens, 1990, p. 28.) If this is so, what can we do about it? He equates modernity with a juggernaut and asks how we can 'harness the juggernaut' of modernity which seems to be out of our control but which we neither should, nor can, give up attempting to steer (Giddens, 1990, p. 151).

Practice implications

What are some of the implications of the incident for my practice as a nurse teacher? Carr and Kemmis suggest that 'Practices are changed by changing the ways in which they are understood' (Carr and Kemmis, 1986, p. 91). This is not necessarily a comfortable process. I was 'acutely' (again!) aware of the impact of the incident in terms of the difficulty in 'getting my act together' at the beginning of a new term as the result of disillusion and questioning, 'what *do* we think we're doing – is there *any* point in it all?' What has happened about the much quoted document 'A Vision for the Future' (Department of Health (DoH), 1993) which devotes a whole page to the topic of 'Individualised Patient Care' and includes reference to meeting patients' and clients' needs 'in collaboration with them, and their carers . . . based on systematic and individual assessment of care needs . . .' (DoH, 1993, 3.13). A number of Charters stemmed from the government's Citizen's Charter: these included the Patient's Charter (Department of Health, 1992, 1995).

The 1992 version includes National Charter Standard 8 which states, 'A named, qualified nurse, midwife or health visitor will be responsible for each patient' (DoH, 1992, p. 15). The 1995 version states, 'You can *expect* a qualified nurse, midwife or health visitor to be responsible for your nursing or midwifery care. You will be told their name.' The next paragraph states that, 'If you agree, you can expect your relatives and friends to be kept up to date with the progress of your treatment' (DoH, 1995, p. 14).

The incident described seemed to illustrate a theory–practice gap somewhere, and as Savage (1995) suggests, writing in the *Nursing Times*, the named nurse concept raises a number of issues. Amongst those issues, she suggests, is the link between the concept and government policy. The Royal College of Nursing (1992) saw it for the opportunities it represented in affirming both the value of nurses to patients and recognition of the initiation of such an approach, already in a number of settings. However, for Savage it also characterises a strategy by the government concerning, for example, cost effectiveness, value for money and individual responsibility. This results in the individual nurse becoming responsible for quality of care and patient satisfaction rather than the Trusts or government. Since only a few nurses have been appointed to the purchasing health authorities, approaches to defining what nurses 'do' and how their work is evaluated will often be determined by non-nurses. It is easy to see how not only the patient but also the nurse may be seen as a 'puppet'. This results, as Savage suggests, in a disempowering of nurses through their loss of control whilst at the same time leaving them accountable for other people's interpretation of the named nurse standards. The possibility that nurses may and perhaps do, find themselves with the dilemma of competing values concerning their role becomes evident. It is then perhaps not surprising if the values held as an individual become compromised in the battle to retain a job and income, in simplistic terms, a roof over one's head.

After the incident, I found marking written papers relating to 'discharge' from hospital, where the 'right' words were used about the importance of good assessment and its contribution to 'good' discharge planning, both upsetting and frustrating. Whilst giving a lecture about Community Care, for which one of the key objectives is 'to make proper assessment of need and good case management the cornerstone of high quality care', I found myself having to resist a surprisingly strong temptation to launch into a 'denunciation' about what seemed meaningless rhetoric. What links might there be between the incident, biographical factors and practice as a teacher?

In practice

Is there something of the converted missionary in me, stemming from a lack of willingness to compromise ideals and other evangelical and clerical influences in my biography, in terms of promoting 'community practice ideals' within the school of nursing? Is that perhaps how some colleagues see it? As with many 'converts' (one only has to think of people who have given up smoking, in health terms!) am I seen to overemphasise, in their terms, its importance? Are there links between my dissociation from some of the narrow hierarchical values implicit in my upbringing and my dissociation from those reflected in many hospital settings? When my father was inappropriately assessed, did my feelings represent an element of self-righteousness and perhaps to some extent did I feel that the incident merely went to 'prove' or justify the need to keep 'flying the community flag' as my community colleagues and I are sometimes accused of doing? Was my frustration justified, ought I to take it up with the local managers under my obligations detailed in the Code of Professional Conduct (United Kingdom Central Council for Nursing, Midwifery and Health Visiting (UKCC), 1992), should I allow it to influence my practice as a teacher, can I avoid it doing so? If I did try to avoid doing so, would it be to deny the very values to which I, and many of my colleagues, subscribe and which I believe to be important to hold on to in the current political and social climate? Who are we, to whom those values are important, though? And as Weber questions, in a lecture about increasing bureaucratisation and rationalisation, what can we do to keep a portion of mankind free 'from this parcelling-out of the soul' (Weber, 1976, p. 362)? This is another phrase which acts as a recurrent refrain in my thinking.

The wider context

Why, then, is the notion of 'flying the community flag' apparently so controversial? From our (community) perspective, the flag being flown in front of us seems to be a much larger one, representing institutional, medically oriented interests as of paramount importance. It all begins to seem incredibly juvenile. And yet, there appear to be echoes of similar conflicts in news reports of events in local council meetings, the House of Commons, the United Nations, illustrating politically influenced differences of opinion based on differing values. At the same time there is currently a very real shift in emphasis, from hospital or institutionally based care to community based care. Surely, therefore, it is important to recognise the implications. Further, most care in the community is provided by families and friends – that is, lay people. What, therefore, are some of the factors influencing the contexts in which such individually significant incidents and events occur?

My father's admission to hospital was, in our terms, under the guise of respite care. However, admission to hospital is a medically controlled event and the word 'controlled' is significant in terms of who makes decisions. To my mother, after the initial relief of having two nights of undisturbed sleep, it seemed as if 'they' had 'taken over', as she described it, and as though she was treated as an 'outsider'. Until his admission, she had played a pivotal role in interpreting my father's wishes and being his advocate. This was something which the district nurses visiting my parents had respected and it had been an integral part of my own experience, when working with clients in community settings. In what I can only refer to as my naiveté, I had expected a partnership approach to be evident in his care. After all, I had read articles and books illustrating such approaches. Thus I experienced almost total disbelief on realising that no account had been taken of the main carer's knowledge, by either doctors or nurses, when trying to build up a picture of his needs – in other words, in assessing his needs, together with their biographical, social and cultural influences. I wondered where the holistic care was, about which we read, and talk, so much?

Views underpinning such an approach are suggested by Florence Nightingale. In her notes, first published in 1860, she writes, in relation to observation, 'the power of forming any correct opinion as to the result must entirely depend upon an enquiry into all the conditions in which the patient lives' (Nightingale, 1969, p. 120). She advises against what might now be referred to as a normative approach, in which generalisations are made, by suggesting that averages 'seduce us away from minute observations' (Nightingale, 1969, p. 124). She also writes of how many men (and some women too) behave as though the 'scientific end were the only one in view' (Nightingale, 1969, p. 125). And this was over one hundred years ago! What is it that in effect 'ring fences' some doctors' and nurses' thinking and interferes with a broader perspective on patient or client needs, in institutional settings? It is almost as though the area surrounding an institution insulates it from the outside world. In the 'institution' where I currently work, on the site of a large general hospital, it is necessary to drive off the public roads, through gateways. There is then an internal ring road surrounding the whole site with most of the car parking being on the opposite side of the road from the main building. Is this symbolic of the insulation to which I referred? And yet it is the patient's/client's home that is seen as an 'isolated and challenging setting' in the Project 2000 Report (UKCC, 1986, p. 52). Who sees what as isolated and challenging?

It almost became a challenge to 'pump' information out of the professional carers. It was forthcoming, in a controlled way, if requested, but was not volunteered. However, it can be difficult for hospital staff to gauge whether or not patients do want to be involved in decisions about their care, in a culture in which such a view is promoted. I found myself wondering if it was supposed that we fitted into the category of not wanting to know or, alternatively, that it was uncomfortable for the professionals to have patient's relatives who *did* want to know what was happening. The way to ascertain this, however, is surely through a skilled holistic assessment and should not be assumed, either way. Florence Nightingale, once more, refers to the harm done by apprehension, uncertainty and other concerns (which may or may not always be true) and how, whilst nurses may be busy thinking of other things, the patient may be internally wrestling with 'his' fears.

The danger of professionals using specialist knowledge as a form of 'domination' is discussed by Campbell. He suggests that knowledge for helping and advising others is never value-free. As examples, he refers to a social worker trying to impose 'what is best' on a person, a nurse using skills which infanticise or depersonalise people and doctors who use professional knowledge to create 'inappropriate dependence' or 'ill-founded faith' (Campbell, 1984, p. 90). He also warns that the 'air of mystery' surrounding professional work can be used 'to conceal . . . inadequate standards'. How often is this the case? With relevance to my choosing to write about a personal experience, Campbell suggests that as doctors and nurses we do not make decisions in isolation but that we are influenced by a whole range of experiences, including our upbringing and professional ethos. Similarly, the knowledge used in helping others to learn is never value-free. The risk, in terms of values, would seem to lie in their denial rather than in their recognition.

The implications of exploring the incident

There are both personal and professional implications in terms of exploring an incident such as the one described. From a personal perspective, there has no doubt been an element of catharsis. One of the 'critical friends', to whom I refer shortly, also raised this issue. However, I would suggest that disconcerting incidents in practice are not free from emotive components and that their exploration is also cathartic. It is 'economical with the truth' to presume otherwise and it takes us back to the earlier discussion concerning subjectivity and objectivity. I vividly remember 'professional' incidents, still with discomfort, which caused great anguish at the time. It just happened that at the time of writing, the experience having, and still having, the greatest impact on my practice was of a more 'personal' nature.

Describing the incident and then making the various links with 'theory-in-the-literature' (Bassey, 1990) has shed further light on my personal theory, on the values and assumptions which underpin my practice and the various factors which have influenced them. These include social and cultural influences such as family, school and work experiences of both a practical and an academic nature. However, many questions have remained unanswered. I usually find challenges are stimulating and enjoyable. Value conflicts are seen as opportunities for exploration of the various factors involved and may involve reflection both at the time and later. However, when difficulties arise, it always seems that they occur when my circumstances at that time are overshadowed by events with echoes from earlier days. In such situations, no matter how much effort may be made to 'apply' behavioural theories or be otherwise self-aware, the 'reality' of past experiences is at the forefront. It is then only in retrospect that it is possible to reflect. And since situations are always unique, there seems to be no magic formula for avoiding the advent of new difficulties.

From both a personal and professional viewpoint, I have come to realise that the promotion of the 'community related' values discussed earlier, seem really to concern person-centred values. These encompass a partnership approach and the taking account of the individual and his or her family, friends and community and the particular context of circumstances, incidents and situations together with the factors which influence them. Such values are fundamental to work with people in their own home but are not always so easily achieved in institutional settings. It has reinforced my resolve to keep such person-centred, humanistic and holistically oriented values as a central focus for students, in my practice as a teacher. My references to published literature help me to 'explore connections' and to go through the process suggested by Oakeshott, to which I referred earlier. I would use the same approach, whether the incident was of a personal or of a professional nature. I suspect that hidden not far below the surface of even supposedly 'professional' incidents is a *person*, trying to make sense of and understand what occurred. This is so often denied and suppressed in the interests of maintaining 'professional' detachment and objectivity.

Different perspectives

I am conscious of the risk of my views becoming uncompromising ideals, particularly at times when tensions arise. Another critical friend observed that there seemed to be 'quite a bit about control' in the chapter. When such tensions arise, am I reacting to and resisting the implied 'control' of myself by others? I wonder how much the 'controlling' influences of my upbringing and the sort of control evident in the hospital setting of the incident, in addition to my 'institutional' work experiences, have a counter effect. Is part of the appeal of work in the community a reflection of my preference to be independent and in control of my activities and to be fully responsible and accountable for them and less under the control of others? Is my strong desire for recognition of people as unique persons, in particular and varying circumstances and not as puppets or mere role performers, yet another manifestation of 'control' but from a different perspective?

Another comment concerned the recurrent theme of 'community'. This is something else on which to reflect. A very 'closed community' upbringing is not dissimilar, in some ways, to the community in hospitals. Has this led to questioning the implicit values in both, testing other 'communities', finding a compatible non-institutional work community with freedom to, yes, be in control of my day-to-day practice and still be part of a community of like-minded practitioners with similar values? And what about an involvement in an intellectual community of thinking? To me, none of this is about behaviour, or performance which meets the standards of prescribed criteria, it is concerned with a multitude of experiences and how, through the meaning we give to them, they shape and continue to shape our thinking and our values and, therefore, the way we would *like* to practice – and the way we *do* practice, which may not always be the same thing.

I hope that I will continue to attempt to develop and improve my often inadequate skills for handling some of the value conflicts which arise from time to time, through a greater awareness of the alternative perspectives and their influences. At the same time, I believe that it is important, in the words of a respected teacher, 'to keep faith with your [my] vision of education'. This last point can be related to the reference, mentioned earlier, to the 'brilliant' help and guidance from a tutor, reported by one of the participants in my research. Both examples support the value of 'critical friendship' in professional development and illustrate the development of personal theory. This is where I would like to acknowledge the helpful comments of my own critical friends, who patiently read this chapter at intervals during its development and whose comments invariably gave a different perspective to one aspect or another.

I believe that the views expressed support the idea that nursing practice and teaching practice are fundamentally 'social practices' as Langford (1985), and the incident described, suggest. This includes recognising that assumptions about the meanings, for those involved, should never be 'taken for granted'. Each interaction, however similar, is always particular in its circumstance and influences and may be seen from a variety of perspectives. It therefore seems naive to believe that we can programme ourselves to always *re-act*, mechanically, in a guaranteed way. However, I do believe that it is possible for increased understanding, gained through reflective and critical enquiry, to enhance our professional judgement of what might not only be 'technically effective action' but also 'ethically enlightened action' in the particular situations in which we find ourselves at any time. The former is potentially achievable but represents Hyland's (1994) 'lowest common denominator' in terms of person-centred care. The latter can place the practitioner in a risk situation since there may be competing values but I believe it offers the opportunity for the development of professional practice.

Also in professional terms, the incident has illustrated the confusions, and some of their consequences, which may arise through situations which are 'taken for granted' by professionals who adopt the role of 'expert' and do not enter into a partnership with their clients – or colleagues. This, to me, again emphasises the importance of a person-centred, rather than a role-, task-, ageist- or condition-centred, approach. If assessment really is to be 'the cornerstone of high quality care', it seems vital that all health care professionals explore the concept in broad terms.

Further educational implications

This is a period when much concern is being expressed that student nurses lack practical (technical) skills, with recommendations that this should be addressed. Equally, recent research also emphasises their ability to learn and to quickly overcome any practical skills deficits. I believe that, in our desire to address this issue, it is important that pre-registration courses do not lose sight of the interpersonal skills implicit in the person- and context-related learning outcomes for the course, which include identification of the implications of 'disease, disability, or ageing' not only for the individual but also 'her or his family', appreciation of social, political and cultural factors relating to health care, 'awareness of values and concepts of individual care' and to 'conduct therapeutic relationships with patients and clients' (UKCC, 1989).

At post-registration level, the English National Board for Nursing, Midwifery and Health Visiting (ENB) (1990) has described ten Key Characteristics considered to be desirable for practitioners 'working closely with patients and clients'. Key Characteristic Four requires practitioners to 'Use interpersonal skills effectively in relating to team members, clients and carers' and to 'Encourage the contribution of client and carer in the team'. In relation to the incident, there is clearly a need to translate rhetoric into reality. However, it is important to recognise not only the factors which influence personal contexts but also to take account of the historical, cultural, ethical and political factors which influence the contexts within which health care occurs.

Conclusion

Writing in the way illustrated in this chapter challenges the style conventionally expected in nurse education, namely, exploring literature ('theory') pre-judged as relevant for its 'application' to practice. Such an approach leads to practice becoming secondary to theory. It has reinforced my belief (my personal theory) that we should, conversely, encourage students to discuss and to write about practice issues which then lead to the exploration of relevant theory-in-the-literature (Bassey, 1990). Such writing requires theoretical assessments to be grounded in practice using a more creative, less rule following, approach in terms of thinking. It gradually becomes structured in the process of its development. Excerpts from reading are remembered as having relevance to the description and begin to create a 'picture' with depth and substance. I believe that this should incorporate reflection and systematic critical analysis about the particular events or situations, including how they affect the writer, with the first person being used where it is relevant. It is not, however, without implications for challenging traditional values implicit in the structure of the organisation, which is not always a comfortable process. Assessment of theory would complement assessment of practice rather than both apparently being seen as separate issues. Separation of practical and academic work promotes the theory–practice or, more relevantly, the practice–theory gap. Another vitally important professional issue involves the nature of the paradigms and methods chosen for research (and teaching about research) 'to improve and develop practice' within practice settings.

At the beginning, I wrote that I would not use a reflective model for reasons which I hoped would become apparent. I believe that to have done so would have been reductionist, with the emphasis on the model determining the nature of the exploration. The approach used in this chapter, enabling me to explore this particular incident, is based on a broad framework concerning personal, social and professional contexts and some of the factors which influence them. For me, it further illustrates the complicated process of unravelling complex situations and the implications which not only 'professional' incidents can have for our practice.

Reference to the variety of published works which help me to understand the issues relating to the incident, as I see them, has helped me to illustrate further the wide-ranging complexities of the incident and its implications. Many of the references reflect a particular community of thinking, one to which, as I indicated earlier, I am continually aspiring to subscribe because it is the one which I most value. I find it reassuring to discover support for these views from people who have far greater skill than I, in terms of the choice of words to express their thinking.

I believe that writing reflectively and attempting to analyse critically the various aspects of an incident can illustrate how its complexities and confusion can gradually be understood in relation to the various contexts and the factors influencing them. However, this can only be in so far as it is viewed at a particular time. The increased understanding which occurs also raises more questions and the interpretation given to the incident now may be different later, after further reflection. This chapter may have reached the end, in terms of writing, but in terms of thinking it can only represent a provisional understanding of what may never be completely understood.

References

Bassey, M. (1990). On the nature of research in education (Part 1). *Research Intelligence, 36*, 35–38.

Blumer, H. (1969). *Symbolic Interactionism: Perspective and Method.* Prentice Hall.

Campbell, A. (1984). *Moderated Love: A Theology of Professional Care.* SPCK.

Carr, W. and Kemmis, S. (1986). *Becoming Critical: Education, Knowledge and Action Research.* Falmer Press.

Department of Health. (1992). *The Patient's Charter.* HMSO.

Department of Health. (1993). *A Vision for the Future: The Nursing, Midwifery and Health Visiting Contribution to Health and Health Care.* Department of Health.

Department of Health. (1995). *The Patient's Charter and You*. HMSO.

Dewey, J. (1970). *Educational Essays* (J. J. Findlay, ed.), Cedric Chivers (first published 1910).

Dewey, J. and Dewey, E. (1915). *Schools of Tomorrow*. J. M. Dent and Sons.

English National Board for Nursing, Midwifery and Health Visiting. (1990). *A New Structure for Professional Development for Continuing Professional Development and the ENB Higher Award for Nurses, Midwives and Health Visitors*. ENB.

Fish, D. (1989). *Learning Through Practice in Initial Teacher Training: A Challenge for the Partners*. Kogan Page.

Fish, D. and Purr, B. (1991). *An Evaluation of Practice Based Learning in Continuing Professional Education in Nursing, Midwifery and Health Visiting, Project Paper Four*. English National Board for Nursing, Midwifery and Health Visiting.

Giddens, A. (1990). *The Consequences of Modernity*. Polity Press.

Golby, M. (1992). Essay Notes. Reflective Professional Practice. B.Phil./M.Ed. in Professional Studies. University of Exeter (unpublished).

HM Government. (1992). *The Citizen's Charter*. HMSO.

Hyland, T. (1994). *Competence, Education and NVQs. (National Vocational Qualifications) Dissenting Perspectives*. Cassell.

Langford, G. (1985). *Education, Persons and Society: a Philosophical Enquiry*. Macmillan.

Mead, G. H. (1962). *Mind, Self and Society*. University of Chicago Press (first published 1934).

Nightingale, F. (1969). *Notes on Nursing: What it is, and what it is not*. Dover Publications (first published 1860).

Oakeshott, M. (1975). *On Human Conduct*. Clarendon Press.

Pearson, A. (1991). Taking up the challenge: the future for therapeutic nursing. In *Nursing as Therapy* (R. McMahon and A. Pearson, eds.), pp. 192–210. Chapman and Hall.

Peterson, A. D. C. (1957). *Educating our Rulers*. Gerald Duckworth.

Queen Victoria. (1870). Queen Victoria's letter to Sir Theodore Martin, 29 May 1870. In *Oxford Dictionary of Quotations* (1953). Book Club Associates/Oxford University Press.

Royal College of Nursing. (1992). *Issues in Nursing and Health (14). The Named Nurse: Implications for Practice*. London: RCN.

Savage, J. (1995). Political implications of the named-nurse concept. *Nursing Times*, **91**, 36.

Schutz, A. (1964). *Collected Papers II. Studies in Social Theory*. Martinus Nijhoff.

Schutz, A. (1967). *The Phenomenology of the Social World*. Northwestern University Press (first published in German, 1932).

Schutz, A. (1970). *On Phenomenology and Social Relations*. University of Chicago Press.

Schutz, A. (1972). *The Phenomenology of the Social World*. Heinemann Educational.

Thomas, W. I. (1976). The definition of the situation, reprinted from 'The Unadjusted Girl' (The Social Science Research Council). In *Sociological Theory: A Book of Readings* (L. A. Coser and B. Rosenberg, eds.) (4th Edn), pp. 207–209. Collier Macmillan.

United Kingdom Central Council for Nursing, Midwifery and Health Visiting (UKCC). (1986). *Project 2000: A New Preparation for Practice.* UKCC.

United Kingdom Central Council for Nursing, Midwifery and Health Visiting. (1989). *Nurses, Midwives and Health Visitors (Training) Amendment Rules. Rule 18(a), Statutory Instrument 1456.* UKCC.

United Kingdom Central Council for Nursing, Midwifery and Health Visiting. (1992). *Code of Professional Conduct.* UKCC.

Weber, M. (1976). Some consequences of bureaucratization. In *Sociological Theory: a Book of Readings* (L. A. Coser and B. Rosenberg, eds.) (4th Edn), pp. 123–132. Macmillan.

Williams, R. (1976). *Keywords: A Vocabulary of Culture and Society.* Fontana/Croom Helm.

Chapter 6

Dealing with extremes: a personal dilemma

Crissi Gallagher

Introduction

I became involved in writing this chapter as a result of attending a workshop looking at reflective practice run by Della Fish at the University of Southampton School of Occupational Therapy and Physiotherapy in January 1995. At the end of the day, when everyone was packing up and stuffing papers into brief cases, Della invited contributions to a project which was to be aimed at providing health care professional students and practitioners with examples of research using a case study approach and which were centred on reflection and deliberation. My ears pricked and I immediately fancied the idea. Although I had very little information about the task and theoretically should have held back before committing myself, I was more than willing to take up the opportunity. I anticipated that it would be a good personal learning experience to participate in the reflective process and would provide opportunity for me to practise what I preached to students and supervisors. The possibility of publishing my work was also attractive, as this is a high priority for lecturers in a university setting.

The chapter describes an experience I had as co-ordinator of a post-registration programme for newly qualified occupational therapists. I look at a particularly difficult time in the development of the programme, when my personal needs and the needs of the programme came into conflict. I reflect on this experience at different stages over a period of months and identify what I learnt about myself and the programme, in both the short and long term. I have attempted to structure the reflection into immediate, intermediate and final stages, but last minute observations and insights are included under 'Stop Press' headings and present my most up to date personal reflections.

Background to the critical incidents

I worked as education co-ordinator for Southampton Occupational Therapy Services and had several years' experience of co-ordinating post-registration programmes for newly qualified therapists recruited to the service. The programmes ran annually from September to October of the following year. Having worked with many newly qualified therapists (participants) in this way I was confident in my ability to provide positive educational experiences in such pro- grammes. I believed, rightly or wrongly, that I had a reasonably good understanding of participants' needs and aspirations. However, the 1993–1994 post-registration year was to prove exhausting.

The two day introductory workshop provided me with an insight into the participants' needs and set the pace for the rest of the programme. I quickly recognised that, although some participants were prepared to meet me half way in this process, a small number who knew each other well, having trained together, were already forming into an unco-operative sub-group. They obviously had a very different agenda from mine and the other participants. They talked loudly amongst themselves, giggled throughout most of the dialogue and related everything to their negative experience of training. An awkward and increasingly uncomfortable situation was developing.

In fact they disrupted the workshop so much that I was left with little choice but to forget the planned timetable, think on my feet and give them opportunity to talk at length. I judged that it was a risk worth taking and one which I initially hoped to contain within this workshop. They discussed their lasting perceptions of training and provided vivid examples of poor teaching and lack of support and feedback. Although I was surprised at their limited level of understanding and appreciation of the learning opportunities now on offer I hoped that allowing them 'air time' would throw new light on their past experiences and enable them to make a more constructive start. Eventually I began to pick up signs that although the other participants listened and offered comments as best they could, they were becoming increasingly impatient to learn more about the programme and to move on at a faster pace. I attempted to strike an uneasy balance between the opposing needs of the two groups but it was obvious that this was an impossible task. As the year progressed this conflict of interest continued. I knew that ideally I should split the group into two but this was not a realistic or feasible option. I felt constrained to carry out the programme as agreed with managers and senior therapists within the service, so I opted to continue with the schedule and hoped to build up participants' confidence and gain their co-operation along the way.

They challenged me and the programme constantly in a way which slowly eroded any chance of negotiating a needs-led approach. For example, early on in the programme a Time Management module got off to a poor start when participants arrived at 9.00 a.m. and the tutors arrived at 9.30 a.m. to face an angry group who felt that their time had been wasted. The schedule clearly stated a 9.30 a.m. start, but there seemed little point in referring to this. They appeared to relish putting tutors in their place, but were not ready to use this responsibility constructively in a mature manner. Written feedback on subsequent modules further emphasised the different needs; for example, half the group would value a workshop while the other half felt it was rubbish. Some comments were particularly vicious and unproductive, which resulted in a no-win situation.

Throughout the process I never doubted the decisions that I made, to administer the modules in the usual way and to expect participants to make their own choices about the modules they would attend. However, it became increasingly difficult to live with the consequences of these judgements on a personal level.

A critical incident

In July I was summoned to join their peer group to discuss the programme. I listened for the best part of an hour to the long list of complaints about the programme and my shortcomings as co-ordinator. When the ring leaders presented me with a list of work-shops undertaken in another district and childishly demanded to know why they did not have the same provision, my patience finally snapped. If they had shown any interest in anything other than themselves they would have realised that all members of staff had access to a very comprehensive programme held within the service. It was obvious that they had not grasped the training situation correctly and I suggested that they get the facts right before they complained in future. When they realised they had made a silly mistake in not checking their facts this somehow incensed them further.

While one or two embarrassed participants tried to retrieve their dignity and placate the situation, I was forcibly struck with how little they had all developed over the past months. I felt disinclined to take the criticism any longer. For a moment I gave up acting as the co-ordinator and said what I felt, instead of what should be said. I queried whether they had ever stopped to think about how the situation made me feel, and what it was like to be the butt of their hostility and lack of co-operation over such a long period of time. There was a short uncomfortable silence, one or two guilty looks and a lot of fidgeting in seats. By introducing a personal context into the situation I had silenced them momentarily, but I knew this would not alter anything in the long term. They still were not able to present their suggestions in a constructive way, and I finally realised that I must accept defeat. I was annoyed with myself for giving up, disappointed with their lack of progress and very glad that the year was coming to a close.

A critical meeting

The newly appointed Director of Occupational Therapy Practice (DOTP) in Southampton Community Health Service NHS Trust was concerned about feedback she had received about the programme from heads of departments and myself as co-ordinator. She decided it was time for a re-think and a meeting was organised in October between representatives from all the Occupational Therapy Departments across the service. I realised that anyone in a new post is likely to want to review the situation. However, I still felt that I was in a particularly vulnerable situation as I was not really sure what the purpose of the meeting was or what would be brought up, and I found this quite threatening. Obviously something had been mentioned by the heads of departments that I was not aware of and which put me at a disadvantage.

In the space of an hour and a half a group of nine senior therapists, who had experience of working with and supervising participants on the 1993–1994 programme or teaching specific modules, discussed the programme and identified how it might be developed in the future. We met in a large, unfamiliar conference room across a large conference table and ceremonially took it in turns to put our cards down on the table.

The DOTP welcomed everyone to the meeting and invited me to open the discussion by sharing my experience of working with the 1993–1994 group of twelve participants. I tried to summarise the situation that had developed over the year, reporting that the participants had many positive individual attributes, but they were a difficult and demanding group. I felt compelled to explain how I had tried everything within my experience and ingenuity to cope with the negative nature of their demands without much success. I tried to cover this in as unemotional a way as possible, which was difficult as the programme had not quite finished and I was still in 'survival' mode.

I felt that brevity was important and tried not to dwell for long on the difficulties of the particular group. However, it was a useful way of setting the scene and one or two supportive comments were shared along the lines of, 'I also found ... very difficult to supervise, there was no pleasing her', or, 'if you found them difficult, then they must have been bad!' I believe that there were one or two people in the meeting who could commiserate with me in the light of their own experience of specific participants, but that the others really did not understand how traumatic it had been. However, for a brief moment I basked in positive peer support and felt much better.

Each course participant had been supervised by a senior therapist, on a one-to-one basis, within the workplace throughout the year. As co-ordinator of the programme it was part of my role to meet with these supervisors on a regular basis. I reported that I had spent more time supporting these supervisors over recent months than in the previous six years because of the pressure they had felt from participants. The fact that some participants had been difficult in the clinical situation seemed to be a useful indicator of just how 'bad' they had been. I remember putting this issue forward quite forcefully as it was reassuring that my judgement of the situation was supported by others.

After a short time we began to brainstorm how we might develop the programme in the future. It was our normal practice to review the programme but on this occasion I felt that we were over-reacting and were being driven by the anxiety created by the 1993–1994 participants instead of planning in our usual way. I was angry to think that this group had such influence on the proceedings. In fact the discussion became more animated only when, freed from thinking about them, we were able to put forward new ideas and suggestions. Then everyone, including myself, got carried away with the discussion and became enthusiastic about scrapping the old and bringing in the new. Although I agreed with all the ideas and found them exciting, in the back of my mind I kept thinking, "that's fine but how on earth can this be implemented?"

The overall tone of the discussion was 'let's throw away everything we've done in the past, it hasn't worked'. As I had worked hard on the programme over the years, it was difficult to take any criticism without feeling personal about it. I chose to control my frustration rather than share it even though I was 'put out' because it appeared that members of the meeting were more prepared to take the participants' negative view rather than supporting me.

I listened to the discussion for about fifteen minutes, though it seemed much longer. I felt a need to dissociate myself from the conversation, and was surprised to hear myself saying, "that's a good idea, how do you suggest we carry this out?", while in my head I was thinking, "I don't believe this, where do I start? They don't know what this means." I couldn't say this without sounding negative, which I was determined not to do.

I felt similarly out of control at this stage of the meeting and there was a gigantic battle going on inside me about the right thing to do in the circumstances. It was extremely hard not to sound defensive when the programme was being taken apart or criticised. I felt that my judgement was on the line. After my initial introduction I remember listening a lot and not saying as much as usual. I couldn't trust myself to speak or to resist the desire to say "been there" and "done that". As there was a lot to cover and everyone had quite a lot to say, I don't think that my 'quietness' or personal struggle was noticeable to anyone but myself.

Eventually we decided on the essential components of the programme, which appeared to me to be essentially the same as those offered in previous years, apart from the introduction of a personal and professional portfolio process which would encourage individual autonomy. This appeared to be a satisfactory compromise as, while retaining some stability in content, it allowed us to build on and develop existing resources.

I agreed to mould the ideas into something practical, even though in reality the time scale was (seemed) impossible. It was a challenge and somewhat gratifying that the group trusted me to carry out their ideas. Members of the meeting appeared to feel better having put their point of view forward, the meeting was closed and everyone went on with their business, leaving me to do the work! I wondered what would have happened if I had not volunteered to do the re-organising, but more importantly, how I would have felt if I had not been allowed to take back control of the situation.

Immediate reflections on the critical incidents

Normally I try to embrace new ideas and creative thinking with enthusiasm, but this was definitely not how I felt about this situation. I found it hard to differentiate between what was best for the programme and what was best for me. I needed to understand this before I could get on with the work, so I spent a week or two after the meeting reflecting on the experience. Interestingly, my reflections centred around my feelings about the participants rather than the meeting itself, though it had acted as a catalyst to make me stop and think before I put anything into action.

My relationship with the participants influenced every decision I made and everything I did. I desperately wanted to embrace new ideas, but I was mortified by the idea that they would think that any radical changes had come about purely because of their influence. They did not deserve to have this sense of achievement and I could not bear the thought of giving them this satisfaction, when in fact some of the proposed changes had been under consideration for much longer. When I look back on this I realise just how damaging a group they had been from my perspective, and working with them for the whole year had affected me more than I had imagined.

Boud et al. (1987) discuss the importance of taking into account the affective components of learning and how teachers can only have access to what the students choose to reveal. On reflection I can see how the participants had undermined the programme with their rigid interpretation of the rules and guidelines, which was totally opposed to my more intuitive approach. This was probably the reason for the build up of tension between us throughout the year. I recognised the short term effect of this and dealt with it by letting off steam with trusted peers, but I was surprised that in the long term, many months later, I was still struggling to put it into a workable context.

I understand that my experience as a therapist/educator allows me to develop high level communication skills, at the same time as being able to look at the whole picture (Fleming, 1991). My hopes and aspirations were to build up relationships with participants in order to share skills and experiences, but their apparently blinkered approach to the issues came into conflict with this. I felt that the group's overall approach was immature and short sighted, and was quite procedural in nature, they demonstrated limited reasoning skills when they were together. With hindsight I can see that perhaps this was excusable as they were newly qualified and I could be deemed to have much more experience (Benner, 1984; Yarrett Slater and Cohn, 1991), but at the time it was quite provoking.

I felt responsible for ensuring that everyone's experiences while on the programme were positive, but as I had no control over their previous experiences it was frustrating that I could not help them to move on. They were obviously angry about many things and I worried about the influence this had on the other participants. I tried many times to interact with them, but could not find a shared language. I had never experienced such a large gap in expectations before, or such resistance to closing it. As a result I was carrying a lot of anger, some of it my own admittedly, but much of it was theirs.

Stop Press

I made a mistake in thinking that participants could run before they could walk and tried to get them to discuss their needs, without giving them enough time to reflect on the experience. At first I felt hurt by their rejection, then I too became angry, hence words such as 'mortified, harassed, rigid, blinkered and frustrating'. I appear to have used the literature quite successfully to take this further and vent my frustration by describing them as 'immature, short sighted and procedural' in its most negative sense. When I reflect on this now I am shocked that I was quite so judgemental and can honestly say that I am no longer angry now that I have shed light on the situation. It is true that time and 'reflection' heals.

Comment

All these feelings were compounded because at the time I was split between being a health care practitioner and a university teacher, in two very busy posts. It was the usual scenario of two 'large' halves making more than one whole (which is something that in the health service many people assume is all part of everyday life). I was just about managing with the workload and was seriously considering moving into the university on a full time basis. I felt like a traitor to the health service for even considering this. I really wanted to evaluate and finish all my work, to be able to hand it all over to someone else. The last thing I needed was to be involved in a complete review and overhaul of such a major part of my work, particularly when this was not of my own volition. I was angry that they had managed to put me in this position.

It did not feel comfortable to finish the job on a sour note as it negated all the other good things that had been achieved prior to this. I had invested so much of my time, effort and emotion into the programme that I really wanted to finish on a good note. Fleming (1991) describes the compulsion to make it better so as not to leave a mess and the ability to pull it all together, as an important driving force in the work of an experienced therapist. I was relieved to read this and took comfort that other therapists might feel the same.

In fact the other members of the meeting, who were all senior 'expert' therapists, followed a similar pattern. We needed to be negative about a stressful situation and getting this off our chests allowed us to see things clearly once more. After looking at the whole picture from a slightly different angle, most of the important elements were salvaged, though it was necessary to be positive and package it in a different way. We looked for a way of pulling it all together into a nice tidy package and it seemed that reflecting-on-action enabled us to explore our understanding and re-establish the philosophy behind the programme (Schön, 1995; Smith, 1994).

I was excited by the novelty of introducing a new and necessary dimension to the programme to which I felt very committed, but the tiredness was overwhelming. I could see the challenge looming and my heart sank because I knew that I could not ignore it. As co-ordinator I appeared to be the best person to develop the package, but at the time, on a personal level, I was not a good judge of my abilities and it was difficult to know where to start.

Stop Press

I felt pulled in two opposing directions, the positive and negative sides, and use strong words like 'traitor' to describe myself. My personal commitment was under scrutiny which resulted in me making a poor long term judgement about the participants' needs. I must add in my defence that the situation did not happen overnight, but built up over a period of a year. Towards the end of the year I half believed the complaining participants were right because I felt overwhelmed and lacked confidence. This certainly describes my state of mind during the meeting in October.

The Post-registration Programme after October 1994

I used the following couple of weeks to think about ways of developing the programme. A number of days on the word processor resulted in some fairly comprehensive guidelines for developing a professional portfolio. This time was very productive as I believed that using a portfolio to record meaningful learning experiences would encourage self-development and act as a permanent record and basis for continuous reflection (Walker, 1987); it also seemed like a good answer to the issue of meeting individual needs.

The 1993–1994 and 1994–1995 programmes overlapped, so at the same time as starting the new one I had to finish the difficult one. I saw each 1993–1994 participant individually over the following two months to follow up on their experiences. I found it extremely hard to motivate myself to do this, but I managed to see most of them. Overall this reinforced my belief that on an individual basis they appeared much more positive about their experience.

The 1994–1995 group of six participants restored my faith in myself and the philosophy of the programme. Admittedly, after the previous year they really did not have to be very good to be an improvement, but in fact they were the best group I have ever worked with. In both group and individual work they demonstrated the most advanced reasoning skills I had ever encountered in a group of inexperienced therapists.

It was possible to use my previous experience as a clinician to relate to the issues that arose (to draw for example on strategies for working within a team, or coping with a case load). It was satisfying to revisit my own clinical reasoning skills, but in the capacity of an educator, as described by Higgs (1990). I thoroughly enjoyed working with them and in fact when I left the service to work full time at the university in April 1995 I continued to work with them until the following December. I was pleased to have a bona fide reason for prolonging my departure.

Intermediate reflections on the critical incidents
(My thoughts some months later)

During the meeting I was conscious that a decision needed to be made about whether the programme was to be structured or not, and if so, how this might be organised. I did not wish to develop a 'learning to learn' programme as described by Candy et al. (1987). This would encourage participants to be dependent on the structure and stifle any spontaneity. However, in my experience newly qualified therapists could take months to settle down into their new role, they did not always know what they wanted at first and in many ways they needed structure (for example they needed to be told rather than asked about the date and times of a seminar), to feel comfortable in the early stages. As they grew and developed they were more able to take responsibility for making more decisions for themselves.

In my judgement the content of the current programme was creative and allowed individuals to develop because I had frequently asked for and received feedback about this on many occasions. The 1993–1994 group seemed to sabotage every opportunity offered to them, saying that it was not what they wanted. This was a source of great annoyance and disappointment to me and I saw them as prisoners of their rigid competencies (Candy et al., 1987). They may have felt that they had wasted their time but they also wasted everyone else's. I felt I had been imprisoned with them throughout the year, and pushed towards adopting a negative, prescriptive approach.

In my opinion they were not able to take on the required level of responsibility. I became increasingly fearful of relinquishing my control of the group (Rolfe, 1993), which meant that I found it difficult to differentiate between my own need for structure and that of the programme. I became acutely aware of this during the October meeting. Boud *et al.* (1987) suggest that sometimes reflection can be rooted in one fixed perspective at a time when we do not wish to subject all our experiences to the same level of reflective analysis. In some ways this partly excused my behaviour. On one level I enjoyed brainstorming about the programme and where it could go in the future, but as I was not the only contributor to the programme I also felt justified in defending the work and commitment of others. This resulted in a no-win situation.

Stop Press

I seem less emotional in this stage of the reflection as I have had time to gain more control of the situation. The words I use are less dramatic and have a more considered application. Nevertheless this has been an important healing time, and it is only now that I can really begin to unravel what happened and begin to question myself and reflect further.

Final reflections on the critical incidents

The reflective process has helped me to see more clearly how things that happened in my past have shaped and contributed to the way in which I perceive the world (Boud *et al.*, 1987). Having spent some time thinking about this privately, I think that some explanation of my personal theory, for example why I cannot leave things alone and find it hard to finish, might be useful.

Personal and professional development

Me and my family

I come from a working class family, my dad was in the merchant navy and my mum looked after me and my sister single handed for most of the time. We did not relish my dad coming and going so frequently. I can remember occasionally making things for my dad to take back with him as mementoes but most of the time our survival strategy would be to get on with our life as if nothing had happened each time he returned to sea. As a result of this experience I am not very good at finishing things off or bringing things to a close on an emotional level. I am appalling at saying goodbye, particularly when it's someone I'm close to, I never write letters or keep in touch, but when I see the person it's just as if we'd never been parted.

This pattern has also established itself in my working life, which has been spent mainly in Southampton, within the National Health Service. I would get restless after a couple of years and move onto the next clinical challenge, but never so far away that I needed to pack up completely. I could always leave something behind, or keep some element of the work ongoing, a memento, whether it was continuing with a group or providing supervision for the 'new' therapist, or representing the team on a committee. I always manage to send a thank you letter about six months after leaving, which is usually about as long as it takes me to sever my ties and move.

It therefore suited me to have the challenge of changing the programme because it gave me a bona fide reason for maintaining contact. I rose to the challenge and subsequently continued to work with the 1994–1995 programme for eight months after I had actually left the service. This perpetuated my pattern and gave me a tried and tested way of coping with the situation.

My education and work

Why do I find it difficult to ignore a challenge? On reflection I can see another definite pattern in my experiences, and in particular a reaction to feeling, or being told, that I could not do something.

Educationally I was non-descript throughout most of my infant and junior life. I failed my Eleven Plus and went to a Secondary Modern Girls school which was situated in the middle of a rather notorious housing estate. I was not really interested at the time, because as an average student I had very few aspirations.

I do not know whether it is better for an unconfident child to be 'top of a second best school' rather than the 'bottom of the best school', or whether I just rebelled against being put onto the scrap heap, but I blossomed in an amazing way. I was a genuine example of a late developer. Surprisingly I achieved good Ordinary Level and Certificate of Secondary Education examination results and, fired by this success, at sixteen I wanted to have a go at everything at sixth form college. I was advised against doing too much, but after one term was extremely bored, and ended up doing more or less what I had wanted to do in the first place. I was beginning to be a reasonable judge of my own capabilities.

I focused my attention on Occupational Therapy very early, even though the careers adviser tried hard to send me to work in a Cheshire Home, as this would be 'good experience if I wanted to work with people'. I applied late to college but did not get a place so I took a year out to become more independent. When I eventually managed to get there I did not take well to the spoon feeding type of approach that was adopted by the college. My enthusiasm was applauded, but they were not quite sure what I was going to say or do next (a comment from a fieldwork placement report), which made for a very tense situation. I did just enough to conform with expectations, because I could not wait to be let loose to do my own thing. I have been a therapist since 1978, initially finding my niche working with the mentally ill and eventually being drawn towards education.

In 1988 I applied to the university to join a masters course in education. They foolishly did not believe that a health professional would cope with a large group of teachers talking (grumbling) about the introduction of the national curriculum. I reapplied the next year, informing them that perhaps the teachers might learn something from me if they listened. I was notified in January that I had a place and became pregnant in March. Various people asked whether I would put the degree on hold. Undeterred, I attended for the first term in October 1989, had my son in the Christmas holidays and, to the untrained observer, continued with the course as if nothing had happened. I was awarded the degree in 1992.

When the School of Occupational Therapy and Physiotherapy opened in Southampton in April 1992, the question was, did I wish to be a teacher, and if so how could I leave the health service to do this? I had believed that I would always work in the NHS and the mould was hard to break. Some therapists would find this ludicrous, one or two colleagues actually said, "congratulations on your escape!", which is a sad reflection on the pressures that everyone is working under in the health service. In fact I was not too keen to leave my job. I had a lot of autonomy and believed that colleagues valued and trusted me. I worked hard and the role suited me. So in just the same way as I opted to do everything at sixth form college, instead of choosing between the two jobs I tried to do both!

The October meeting was held at a very crucial time for me. I had been working in the split post for over a year, and was fast realising that it was an impossible task for me. Although outwardly I was coping I knew that realistically I could not maintain it for much longer. I was aware that an increase in my hours with the School was possible and the attractions were getting harder to resist. This was a very difficult decision which would have implications for me, my family and work colleagues, so it was not taken lightly.

Reflection on my personal theory

Now that I can distance myself from these experiences, and am not too immersed in the feelings, I realise that I am no longer happy to be the average student. This reflection-on-action gives me powerful insight and confidence (Cross, 1993; Smith, 1994). Replaying the incident and actually recording it has allowed me to pull together some of the reasons for my reaction and I begin to understand why I am driven to take on a challenge when I see one. The more impossible it seems, the more likely I am to have a go for my own satisfaction, as long as it is on my terms. There have been too many times in the past when I have wasted time as a result of other people's decisions about me, hence my comments on whether I was a good judge of my capabilities, and I know myself well enough to justify my impatience.

However, this does not counteract the constant battle between how I feel inside, which is feeling unconfident about doing something, and at the same time knowing that I really can do it. I find I am almost dependent on someone questioning whether I can do it in order to galvanise me into action. People who know me well rarely suggest that I cannot do something, which means that I am forced into doing this for myself more and more often. Ironically I actually feel less confident in some areas because of this. I find this innate self-doubt very irritating.

Stop Press

I am struck yet again by the way I feel pressured to be a good judge of myself and situations when in fact, like many other people, this judgement varies according to the situation. The most important factor is that I need the opportunity to make up my own mind without interference from others. I appear always to be dealing with extremes, such as the 'top or bottom', 'positive or negative', which feels like a 'gigantic battle' ground and leads me onto the next focus of my reflection.

Technical rational versus creative artistic characteristics

At one point during the October meeting I felt confused and out of control. There seemed to be two very strong forces driving me. I was attempting to rationalise and control my negative feelings about the 1993–1994 participants without much success. I found this struggle inhibited my normal positive approach to working with the people around me.

Looking back to work I did in the early 1980s with colleagues who were working on a therapeutic day hospital (mental health), where we looked at Jung's (1964) theories and explored symbolism, I can vividly remember the symbol of an overflowing cup and my fruitless attempts at catching all the wasted water. I understood this to mean that due to a lack of personal control I had an abundance of wasted creative energy. Similar to anyone else who was fearful of being different from the crowd (Rubenfeld and Scheffer, 1995), I felt that being creative meant being unpredictable, therefore, creativity was a weakness which must be overcome at any cost if I was to appear as skilled as others in the multi-disciplinary team. The term professional artistry was not part of my vocabulary at this time and over the next few years I worked hard to channel and control my time and creative energy into a more acceptable package.

This issue of control suddenly re-surfaced during a discussion about the technical and artistic point of view in Della's January 1995 workshop and as a result of reflecting on my critical incident I began to unravel some of the issues. I found a useful explanation of this in Fish (1991). I find evidence of both in my approach and am aware of a conflict of interest that occurs as a result of trying to control the creative aspect in a logical rational way.

There are many examples where I sit comfortably in the technical rational model. For instance I find the bureaucratic and behavourist approach of National Vocational Qualifications acceptable and am a qualified assessor in this system. I am at ease with the concepts of assessment, appraisal and accreditation, as the structure is productive as well as being reassuring. However, I also believe that personal and professional activity is more than a technical skill. I am constantly interpreting and appreciating my actions and experiences in a reflective way that sits comfortably in the professional artistry model as described by Fish (1991).

I find that I incorporate and combine both models in my everyday work. For instance, I am willing to devote many hours to carrying out intensive video workshops where participants reflect on their performance, but feel compelled to produce a handbook full of theories and information to back this up. Or when attempting to capture the essence and creativity involved in a fieldwork supervisor–student relationship I produce an accreditation document based on logical structured standards.

This trait is also apparent in the way I structure undergraduate and postgraduate teaching sessions, where I concentrate on the development of personal reflective skills and automatically produce structured workbooks and handouts for every session. I would like to believe that I usually provide this background information because I recognise that learners who are functioning at a novice or advanced beginner stage will benefit from this structure, which is a positive side of being an experienced teacher (Benner, 1984). However, there are times when I feel this verges on a more negative need for control and organisation, as in the case of the 1993–1994 postgraduate programme, and I find this mixture quite perplexing.

For me the technical and artistic approach are closely bound together into a very exhausting package. I find I am drawn to therapists who are similar, or have the capacity to be both. If someone has a bias for one or the other I find them much more difficult to relate to and handle, but I also envy their apparently easier and less complicated life style.

Stop Press

This area of conflict has been the most difficult to write about, though I must admit that reflecting on it has increased my understanding and reduced the muddle and intensity of my feelings about it. Obviously being part of the National Health Service for many years has meant that I have become accustomed to a bureaucratic approach, though as a therapist/clinical teacher I have always placed emphasis on professional judgement and personal reflection as well. Therefore I am a product of both types of experiences. They are a part of me and account for my thoughts and actions.

Having discussed this with my peers and regained confidence in my own abilities I begin to feel that my need to control things (a technical rational trait), and my need to participate actively in events (a professional artistry trait), thus partaking of both models, is a strength rather than a weakness. Since I am dealing with extreme forces, which are sometimes in opposition, as in the case of negative and positive elements, perhaps there is something electric and powerful about my approach!

Reflecting on the reflective process

Collaboration with other contributors

Boud *et al.* (1987) highlight how there are limits on what a person can do unaided, and how learning from experience can be accelerated by appropriate support and encouragement from others. This exactly describes the experience of working with the group of contributors to the book, and how we inspired and motivated each other on an individual level.

In our group meetings we discussed many important theoretical and personal issues, but no sooner had I got a reasonable handle on the subject, than something else would be introduced which would confuse me yet again. There were so many dimensions that I felt I would never get to grips with it all. I panicked a little when others seemed to be further on than me but overall this spurred me on to make a start and I began to gain insight into the process through listening to others in the group come to terms with it. In this way we drew on personal and professional experience, and shared different interpretations of events.

Working alongside others I began to realise that although there were great differences in our approaches we shared the stress of coping with large workloads in clinical and educational settings. I could have spent a lot of time wondering why others seemed to be better able to cope with specific stages than me, in, for example, writing up and finishing the task. However, early on in the discussions it became obvious that the process I was going through needed to be unique to me and I began to feel more comfortable. It became less and less relevant to compare myself with others and more interesting to share the issues. It seemed appropriate that some members should be more proficient at some things than others and it was noticeable that we all had different strengths and weaknesses. The collaborative element has been a very powerful learning experience.

This was particularly apparent for Judith (Chapter 9) and me, as we work in the same school and actually teach undergraduate and postgraduate students together. Each of us had a completely different starting point and critical incident, but we enjoyed the luxury of assisting each other through the different stages. Being able to share knowledge and experiences along the way was a riveting and powerful experience. We were able to reflect together on shared practical experiences, such as running a module, or participating in an in-house workshop. We observed each other in action, provided instant feedback and noticed subtle changes in approach and practice.

Writing up the experience

It took me half an hour to decide on the memorable critical incidents, months to reflect on them, and many relentless hours to write them up. Mattingly (1991) describes my plight very well when she suggests that 'words always fall short of practice'. My Yorkshire background and cultural influences are strong, as is my tendency to be open and outspoken, but grammatically I sometimes cannot find the correct words to explain the way I think and speak.

Although I recognise the components of reflective thinking and can teach others about reflective practice, explaining this on paper is a different matter. I tend to read a situation from professional practice rather than theoretical knowledge, I investigate from practice (Munroe, 1995; Schön, 1995). I can come up with ideas, and very occasionally these flow in a coherent fashion onto the paper, but there is a tendency to brainstorm rubbish and spend long hours making sense of it all at a later date. Often I found myself stopping the car in order to write down something profound before it was forgotten. I also often needed to leave it for a few days so that I could approach it with renewed vigour and insight. I worked in fits and starts because the situation was so intense that I could not possibly maintain it consistently.

Early on in the process I felt quite trapped and de-skilled at the thought of linking my thoughts and experiences to other people's work. I wanted to write my own thoughts first because I worried that I would too easily accept the views of others as I lacked experience (Boud *et al.*, 1987). This was a new experience, as I do not naturally conform to other people's ideas in areas of practice where I am more confident.

While I was preparing for my masters dissertation I discovered a chapter by Stronach (1987). His words were deceptively simple, but have had a lasting effect on me. He made me laugh and I related to the scenarios that he mentioned, in particular that you read as little as you can get away with. When I eventually did get around to reading, I overdosed on the information. Everything I read took on a major significance and it was difficult not to apply every paragraph to myself and I had to remind myself to focus on the most important issues. I began to reel from the experience and had this odd feeling that I was drowning in a sea of paper. Although initially I resisted referring to the literature I knew my dissertation could not be finished without it and it was quite tempting to cram in as many references as possible. This time I decided that I would write my thoughts first, followed by a visit to the literature with a more focused approach. Either way I found that the initial stages were drawn out at the expense of finishing well and I realise now that consulting the literature on the way through the thinking and writing is most appropriate.

The state of panic I reached as I continually put off the writing up made me feel as if I was waiting to take an exam without knowing what the subject was going to be (Stronach, 1987). It was very difficult to pull everything together, as finishing is not one of my strengths. I could create the links and organise the material but I simply was not disciplined enough to get down to writing it. I came up with a variety of interesting strategies for procrastinating. Contrary to the perception that lecturers have time to do these 'academic' things, most of the writing has been carried out in my own time, in the evenings or at weekends, so my family were also affected by this commitment.

But I slowly realised that I was expecting to be proficient at writing where in reality I was a novice or at most an advanced beginner, because I lacked experience. I did not have the benefit of this insight until very late in the process, but I know that in the future I will look back on this and be able to place it in a better perspective.

Stronach (1987) suggests that 'there can be experts on evaluation, but never expert evaluators'. I now realise that this applies even when the subject is yourself. There is little chance of thinking about every angle or of really being an expert in every experience. Writing up has been the greatest struggle, but I have enjoyed taking the opportunity to do it and to have a final product at the end. Perhaps it is unrealistic for me to aspire to be an expert without carrying out an apprenticeship.

Stop Press

Ironically, at a time when I should be concentrating on finishing things I am constantly starting new things. I also recognise that every now and then over the years I have had small spurts of activity that bear little relationship to the priorities of the time, which seem to act as a pressure release and lift the lid I have put on my creativity.

Final reflection on the learning process

During March 1996 I shared this chapter with my mother, and the one memorable comment she made was, "You are many things but you are not organised." Despite myself, I thought about this for some time. She's right, I'm not organised, in fact I had filed my articles and references for this chapter so inefficiently over the months that when I was under pressure and needed them I was let down.

As a creative and artistic person I actually need to be more disciplined than organised. I enjoy creating and making the links, but on my own terms. I struggle with writing because the system says I must do it and I instantly fight against this. It is not that I cannot do it. I knew I would struggle to represent my thoughts on paper. Boud *et al.* (1987) highlight how the conventions of professional writing decree that single personal examples are not an appropriate subject, and that because of this, somehow, personal experience has been devalued in the quest for work that is generalisable and objective. Yet even in writing personally *I feel deskilled because unfortunately I am not really able to demonstrate the true extent of my learning because of limitations in my use of language and grammar.* To compensate for this apparent lack of skill I devoted extensive time and energy to this project because I believed in its effectiveness on a personal level.

Stop Press

When I wrote that I believed it. I now think that if I have a clear understanding of an issue I can explain it. What I have to accept is that others might think and write differently.

Comment

Boud *et al.* (1987) state that to teach is to learn twice, to experience a double delight. As teaching is currently my equivalent to clinical work I am in a fortunate position of setting up learning situations which introduce students to the reflective process. I am keen not to adopt traditional teaching and learning methods, preferring to stimulate a higher level of problem-solving (Barker Schwartz, 1991). Offering students real opportunities to learn how to reflect on their experiences and providing them with tools to do this is quite a challenge. It is quite clear to me that my current reflective experience has influenced my approach to developing teaching sessions, which can now be realistic, based in practice not just theories. I understand their struggles and am more patient than in the past.

Stop Press

This was my opinion less than a month ago, but having just marked a number of students' reflective reports, I question whether I am more patient. It is particularly disappointing when students are unable or unwilling to reference their stories. Perhaps this is a case of 'if I have made the effort, why can't you'. I am much more confident (or cut throat) about failing a student who does not meet the requirements. Is this fair judgement or am I expecting them to do what I cannot? I will need to think about this before putting it into a proper context.

Comment

I am able to live with risk and uncertainty and become impatient with people who play it safe. I strive to be able, clearly and critically, to analyse the reasons for my decisions and actions as a way of developing my knowledge base. This appears to confirm the suggestion made by Parham (1987) that the more experienced therapist puts greater value on development and understanding theories. Boud *et al.* (1987) suggest that an original idea can be re-shaped by later reflection and a fuller interpretation. I have re-visited past experiences and perceptions from a more recent point of view and find that gaining a greater understanding of my strengths and weaknesses makes it easier to visualise how I can adapt and be more flexible in future learning situations. In doing so I believe I have travelled some way towards accepting myself as I am. The critical incidents acted as catalysts for change and I recognise the need to continue reflecting on my performance. This self-exploration exercise has helped me to identify strategies that will assist me to become a good university worker. I have told my story in the hope that some of the issues raised could be of interest to others who work in staff development within the health service and because I believe that readers might be able to relate to the conflict of personal and professional issues that I have experienced.

Stop Press

I am having difficulty in detaching and bringing this chapter to a close. Identifying one or two single critical incidents has helped me to explore some very complex issues in an interesting and progressive way. But I must remember Stronach's (1987) words, that there will always be in any investigation questions that were ignored or inadequately addressed, but that there is 'almost always a next time'. I wish you success in your reflective journeys.

References

Barker Schwartz, K. (1991). Clinical reasoning and new ideas on intelligence: implications for teaching and learning. *American Journal of Occupational Therapy*, **45**, 1033–1037.

Benner, P. (1984). *From Novice to Expert. Excellence and Power in Clinical Nurse Practice*. Addison-Wesley.

Boud, D., Keogh, R. and Walker, D. (1987). *Reflection: Turning Experience into Learning*. Kogan Page.

Candy, P., Harri-Augstein, S. and Thomas, L. (1987). Reflection and the self-organised learner: a model of learning conversation. In *Reflection: Turning Experience into Learning* (D. Boud, R. Keogh and D. Walker, eds.), Kogan Page.

Cross, V. (1993). Introducing physiotherapy students to the idea of 'reflective practice'. *Medical Teacher*, **15**, 293–307.

Fish, D. (1991). But can you prove it? Quality assurance and the reflective practitioner. *Assessment and Evaluation in Higher Education*, **16**, 22–36.

Fleming, M. (1991). The therapist with the three track mind. *American Journal of Occupational Therapy*, **45**, 1007–1014.

Higgs, J. (1990). Fostering the acquisition of clinical reasoning skills. *New Zealand Journal of Physiotherapy*, **12**, 13–17.

Jung, C. (1964). *Man and his Symbols* (Illustrated Edition). Aldus Books.

Mattingly, C. (1991). What is clinical reasoning? *American Journal of Occupational Therapy*, **45**, 979–986.

Munroe, H. (1995). Perspective on clinical reasoning. *British Journal of Therapy and Rehabilitation*, **2**, 313–317.

Parham, D. (1987). Toward professionalism: the reflective therapist. *American Journal of Occupational Therapy*, **41**, 555–561.

Rolfe, G. (1993). Towards a theory of student-centred nurse education: overcoming the constraints of a professional curriculum. *Nurse Education Today*, **13**, 149–154.

Rubenfeld, M. and Scheffer, B. (1995). *Critical Thinking in Nursing: an Interactive Approach*. J. B. Lippincott.

Schön, D. A. (1995). *The Reflective Practitioner. How Professionals Think in Action*. Arena Publishing.

Smith, M. (1994). *Local Education. Reflection-in-action.* Open University Press.

Stronach, I. (1987). Practical evaluation. In *Evaluating Education: Issues and Methods* (R. Murphy and H. Torrance, eds.), pp. 204–212. PCP Education Series.

Walker, D. (1987). Writing and reflection. In *Reflection: Turning Experience into Learning* (D. Boud, R. Keogh and D. Walker, eds.), pp. 52–68. Kogan Page.

Yarett Slater, D. and Cohn, E. S. (1991). Staff development through analysis of practice. *American Journal of Occupational Therapy,* **45,** 1038–1044.

Chapter 7

Good practice: lessons in working together

Richard Hillier

Introduction

I am a consultant physician in palliative care, a medical specialty
better known to the lay public as 'hospice medicine'. I qualified at
St Bartholomew's Hospital in London in 1964, and after two years'
surgery changed to medicine, where I felt much more at home. I
then had an opportunity to join the Medical Research Council
(MRC) Laboratories in Hampstead, as an MRC Fellow, where I
stayed for five years. During this time I spent eighteen months in
Antarctica, working on human physiology and acclimatisation, a
topic which was very much in fashion at the time, as we were
exploring how to move the military rapidly between different time
zones or between countries with high and low temperatures,
without jeopardising their physical and mental performance. The
work was stimulating and enjoyable and during my time at the
Medical Research Council, I completed my Doctor of Medicine
thesis.

Unlike my colleagues, I began to miss clinical contact with patients.
Also I was not good enough at research to satisfy my own aspirations in an environment where the quality of research was extremely
high. As I write, I cannot help reflecting that this competitive quality
of mine may not be irrelevant to the theme of this chapter. However,
by this time I was in my thirties and married with three children, so

the idea of going back and starting all over again on the medical ladder was not particularly appealing.

Therefore, because I enjoyed what is now rather loosely termed 'whole patient medicine', I chose to train as a General Practitioner (GP) and joined one of the very first training schemes for GPs in Winchester. After two years' training and two years in Exeter, I moved to Hampshire, where I became part of an excellent group practice in a city and was very happy indeed.

Soon after becoming a general practitioner, it began to become obvious that my skills in controlling pain and other distressing symptoms in patients who were dying was not as good as I would like. My patients suffered far more than was necessary, despite my interest and enthusiasm. I therefore visited St Christopher's Hospice in London in 1973. This world famous hospice had opened five years previously and was already making a small, but impressive impact on the neglected topic of caring for the dying. The visit was a revelation. Not only did I find that many of the problems with which I struggled were more easily solved than I dared to believe, but that even Dame Cecily Saunders did not always obtain a perfect result. Like other readers, the recognition that icons are not perfect stimulates me and gives me the confidence to 'have a go'. This inspired me to read everything that I could lay my hands on and develop my practice in palliative care in the home. Two years later, an advertisement appeared in the British Medical Journal for a Medical Director of the second hospice in the British National Health Service. Dame Cecily wrote to me, suggesting that I apply. To do so was an act of potential professional suicide, but was a chance I was prepared to take. I have worked at Countess Mountbatten House ever since. Those of us who started off new hospices at that time were, by choice or by default, pioneers.

I had spent eighteen months in Antarctica and looking back, I can observe a certain perverse weakness for enjoying a challenge – again indicative of an underlying competitive spirit. After the twenty years in Southampton, the service has grown, the expectations and philosophy of hospice care or palliative care as it is now called, have developed beyond belief, with the result that doctors, nurses and many other professions now accept it as a serious subject. Consequently it is now an accepted part of health care in the United Kingdom, and all over the world. It is against this background that my story emerges.

Countess Mountbatten House

I work at Countess Mountbatten House, at Moorgreen Hospital, Southampton. It has twenty-five beds, a multi-professional team working in the community and a small palliative care team in the adjacent university hospitals. All are engaged in teaching and research. Over a thousand patients are referred each year. Half of these never see Countess Mountbatten House. Of the five hundred that do, half are admitted for symptom control, respite care or the management of complex problems, which cannot be easily managed at home or in hospitals. Originally the beds were the core of the service. Today the beds are the back-up to an out-reach service, which exists to complement and support colleagues, and to improve the confidence and the skills of doctors, nurses and others throughout the health and social services. It is difficult to measure success, but at a very crude level, although approximately 75 per cent of patients would choose to die at home if they could, the reality is that in the United Kingdom, 75 per cent of them actually die in hospital. At Countess Mountbatten House, 75 per cent of those patients who are referred do indeed die at home.

Reflective practice

It may shock readers, but before I met the authors of this book, the words 'reflective practice' meant nothing to me. When I had the invitation to participate and mentioned it to my nurse colleagues, I was surprised to find that most knew about it, some were unashamed enthusiasts for it, and many told me that they 'did it all the time'. It is this last statement that proved a challenge to me. The following story is certainly something I could *not* do all the time. Although ostensibly about a relatively simple clinical situation, reflection reveals it to have much wider implications, which include the challenge and complexities of working with colleagues and how one's own agenda can muddy the waters.

The telling of this story and the implications that it has had and is continuing to have on my practice are immense. For that I owe the patient, his family, my GP colleagues and, above all the editors of this book, a great debt. I now know that reflective practice is not something 'one does all the time'. It is about an attitude of mind, which, once embraced, can never be abandoned.

The story

This is based on a real incident, which occurred over a period of a few weeks. You will have your own views as to what was right or wrong. However, more important than this are the feelings that the incident induced. At the time, I did not reflect on this. I experienced them in myself and others and reacted to them automatically.

It may be worth saying here that it is often considered trite to talk about feelings in clinical situations and I acknowledge and recognise that. However, it is the negative and destructive effect of feelings that is the key to this story, yet, once resolved, positive and unexpected outcomes occurred.

The hospital

I was asked to see Peter, aged fifty-five, who had suddenly developed jaundice. He was rapidly referred to hospital and investigations revealed that he had an advanced cancer of the pancreas. He had been admitted to decide whether or not surgery (the only possibility of cure) could be performed. He also had some abdominal discomfort, but the crucial issue at this time was how he should discuss with his surgeon (who was naturally keen to do everything possible to help Peter), whether or not surgery and/or chemotherapy were the options in Peter's best interest.

Peter's wife, Margaret, was present throughout the interview. A friend of theirs, Jane, arrived. It turned out that she had initiated the referral to myself. Not only was she a friend of Peter and his wife, she was also a friend and colleague of mine for whom I had enormous liking and respect and who has had considerable influence on my own personal development.

Over twenty years I have seen, as patients, the friends and relations of many colleagues and indeed a number of colleagues themselves, so this is not an unusual occurrence. Furthermore, I deal with these situations much less intensely than I did. They and their relatives do much better when I treat them routinely and do not offer any 'special favours', which tends to happen at the outset of one's career. Such favours are almost always a mistake!

Peter, Margaret and I discussed what questions to ask the surgeon; how to judge the advantages and disadvantages of what might be offered and not to be afraid to ask direct questions like "will the operation actually cure me or not", or "will I have complications", and "how long might I have to spend in hospital away from my family?" At the same time, Peter wished to know if his disease was incurable; what would be the likely progress and how would he die. Obviously this is a very sensitive area, but Peter was unusually keen to know all possibilities so that he could put any information he obtained into the context of his, Margaret's and his children's life from both a practical (that is, work) and emotional (that is, life) point of view.

Peter specifically wanted to know whether he would get more pain if he did not have the surgery. Pancreatic pain is not easy to manage, but in our team's hands most patients are rendered pain-free and the remainder are sufficiently well controlled for it not to be a major problem. I vividly remember telling Peter this, although it is a comment which I never made lightly. However, on this occasion the remark was the cause of later tension and difficulties.

Peter and I agreed that as he had a very good relationship with his general practitioner, simple advice from me at this stage would solve the pain problem and that our team need not be involved until his GP sought assistance.

Subsequently, Peter met the surgeon and both agreed that in his case the best option was to have no surgery, no chemotherapy and no radiotherapy, but to focus on his quality of life at home with his family. His disease would be fatal and he would probably live for a few months. Despite this bad news, Peter saw his meeting with his surgeon as very positive. He and the family knew now exactly where they stood. With my reassurance about pain he returned home to make the most of what life was left for him and the family.

The first phone call

About one month later, in the evening, the phone rang. My colleague, Peter's friend Jane, was calling. She explained that she was ringing with Peter's agreement and told a sorry tale of increasingly severe abdominal and back pain, which was causing considerable distress both to Peter and his family. Peter was taking morphine, which reduced his pain for only a short time. It never relieved the pain. She thought that the morphine should be substantially increased. This seemed perfectly reasonable, as well as being safe. Under normal circumstances I would have suggested that they went back to the GP. However, because the situation was escalating and his doctor was not available that weekend, we agreed that the dose should be increased and the GP told as soon as he got back. The other request was that I might review Peter at home.

However, we both knew that as the GP had not formally sought my assistance, this could only happen if the family discussed it with him first. On the following Monday morning I was telephoned by the general practitioner. The family's message had been relayed to him by the practice secretary and he apologised that I had been troubled. He then went on to explain that the situation was now under control and that there was no need for me to be involved. However, he sounded irritated and implied that I had been interfering. He went on to say that he was visiting daily and so was the district nurse. Hence, neither I nor my team were needed. As he spoke, I could feel the tension rising within me. I had clearly overstepped the normal bounds of my practice, if only marginally, and had antagonised the key player (the GP) in the whole situation, making it less likely – not more – that we could be usefully involved in Peter's care in the future. This was a set-back.

I remained convinced that Peter's pain control should be relatively straightforward, if not easy. At best I hoped that this telephone conversation would solve the problem. In practice I was less sure that it would. For although I was saying the right words to the general practitioner and telling him that I was more than happy not to be involved, the GP may well have sensed the feelings of frustration in my voice. Non-verbal messages can be transmitted over the telephone.

What could I have said, which would have helped the situation and engendered a spirit of co-operation? Probably not a great deal. Even when I stick to my own rules of not becoming involved unless formally requested by a colleague, the outcome is usually no better. Indeed, perhaps in those cases, because there was no 'challenge' about my intervention such as occurred here, problems may have been even worse. However, what is of more concern to me is the future relationship with a GP, when many more patients may be involved. So this incident may have had more deleterious effects in the long term.

Another issue was my personal involvement. After all, this was a relatively simple situation, which I considered easily soluble with today's drugs. Not only did I have a patient and family with whom I had related well, but I was also subconsciously keen to be helpful to my colleague and to be seen to be doing good things. In other words, I was becoming personally and emotionally involved, which is very dangerous. Because of this I was convinced that the physical and possibly emotional problems within the family would get worse. Rightly or wrongly I felt that I could influence that for the better and not being able to do so made me irritated, annoyed and, if I am honest, angry. In my righteous indignation at the time, I was unable to recognise any of this.

With these thoughts and feelings, it is impossible that others would not be picking them up as well. I suspect that feelings on both sides were intense and that professional rivalry was developing. However, the striking feature in this story – as in all similar stories – is that these feelings were implicit and not explicit. They were not obvious to me at the time.

The second phone call

Some weeks later, when Peter's GP was on holiday, his partner rang me. Further problems had arisen.

To my shame, I was intensely relieved. Not only did I know the new partner well, but we also respected one another's skills. Suddenly, for me the whole issue underwent a sea change: from anger and frustration to a constructive and friendly collaboration. Peter was now much worse. He required huge doses of morphine and sedation to control his pain, but remained restless, aggressive and was trying to get out of bed. If the pain was controlled, he was delirious; if the pain was not controlled, he was in agony. I was asked to visit that afternoon and agreed with intense relief and obscene enthusiasm, which masqueraded as compassion. The intense unease I feel as I write this, emphasises what my true feelings were. Reflection can be most uncomfortable.

The visit was arranged and I arrived on the same glorious afternoon and was warmly welcomed by Margaret and their daughter and her fiancé, who quickly left. Margaret explained what had happened, which accorded well with what I had already been told earlier that morning. Peter had just had some morphine, before I arrived, but was still restless, incoherent and was trying to get out of bed.

He was bordering on unconsciousness and Margaret thought he was dying. She explained how his drugs had been increased over the past few days, although he remained restless and confused, sometimes aggressive – all symptoms attributed to uncontrolled pain.

However, the situation was becoming clear. Peter had difficulty passing urine and was intensely constipated – both are well-known causes of agitation and restlessness. If these could be relieved, his symptoms should improve and he would require less, not more, sedation and pain killing drugs. The desperation of the clinical team was obvious. They had visited at least once a day, often twice, for several weeks. What shook me (and impressed me) was how well this was received by Margaret and how grateful she was with the care she had received. Indeed, Margaret saw me as almost irrelevant other than to be grateful for my assistance in Peter's physical problems.

On return to the hospital, I rang my general practitioner colleague explaining what I thought needed to be done. If he did not die that night, he needed an indwelling catheter to keep the bladder empty. But it would be too distressing to attempt to relieve his bowels at this late stage. We therefore discussed his drugs and by what route they should be given and to institute this regime as soon as possible.

Peter survived a further forty-eight hours. The agitation disappeared. The pain was relieved and he died peacefully with his family at home. When I was informed, it was with a feeling of intense relief and almost a feeling of justification that after all, my judgement was correct.

Reflection on the Peter-critical incident

As Peter's story progressed the tangle of events became more complex and, from my own point of view, more emotional. Throughout the tale, a number of surprises occurred. Though perhaps these were less surprises, than set-backs which I tried to resolve. After all, I had seen them before in different garb and in different situations. But the uniqueness of Peter's case was that several of these events came together in one incident and dragged out over several weeks.

The obvious dilemmas which may occur in any clinical situation where one is seeing a friend of a colleague were present in Peter's case, so there was nothing remarkable there. I had been in this situation many times. But here, the dilemmas increased to a climax and culminated in a situation which was unique.

The incident began in what I felt was a good initial interview with Peter and his wife, and at which a tricky situation was resolved. Peter and his surgeon avoided being drawn into a situation where unrealistic hope triumphed over reality and were both able to accept the almost certain futility of further therapy. At the same time, neither Peter nor his wife felt they were being abandoned by the hospital when Peter returned home.

The second dilemma was the telephone call from our mutual friend and my colleague, Jane. My handling of this was slightly different from usual. Being medical, Jane could see what was needed and thought she required my support in enabling it to happen. The un-hoped for, but on reflection, inevitable result was irritation for the GP and an increase in activity in the Primary Health Care team, which was appreciated and may or may not have been effective.

The next critical event in the story was when Peter's doctor went on holiday and his partner, well known to me as we had often worked together, took over the case and identified new things which should be done. We both avoided any comments on the story so far because in medicine one is well aware of the dangers of using what some call the 'retrospectoscope'. It is easy to be wise after the event.

The fourth and final event was Peter's death. Although I know how I felt when he died, I had no way of knowing what others felt. For the family it was possibly a relief for Peter that his suffering was over and a deep sadness at his loss. I guess that cancer has a bad reputation and that the pain and distress which occurred was accepted as 'part of having cancer'. I was probably forgiven for seeking to reassure them about pain when in their eyes it was probably inevitable.

The GP's partner was relieved and grateful. I have no idea what their own doctor felt or thought.

But I was deeply dissatisfied. The illness and the distress could have been made better and I felt unhappy that my misguided thoughts to help had in reality misfired and made the situation worse for Peter and his family.

Personal theory

All of us are prone to situations such as the ones described above. We usually handle these either by keeping it to ourselves or, confidentially discussing it with a colleague we trust. The frequent outcome is a shrug of the shoulders, an affirmation that we did the right thing and that the colleague – classically from 'St Elsewhere's' made a mess of it. As a consequence we learn nothing, do nothing and change nothing. We just hope that it will be a long time before anything like it happens again. There is an undoubted feeling of unease; partly with the situation, partly with the other parties concerned, but also, consciously or usually more unconsciously, a deep inner dissatisfaction at the way we handled the whole situation. That is precisely where I found myself at the end of this story were it not for one thing. A year later, I was asked to be involved in this book and to write a chapter about a critical incident which had affected me. By now I had recognised my serious unease with this story. However, I had no solutions, but felt that an honest reflection about what was going on might be profitable, to me and, I hope, to readers. This gave me the opportunity to stand back and observe the story from the outside with the advantage that some time had elapsed since the incident had occurred.

Now I appreciate that many readers will see all the faults, all the solutions and as a result, flip through this chapter eagerly to get on to the next. What I would like to emphasise is that for *me* this was and remained a real dilemma and the more I looked at it the more I saw deep personal feelings, many unconscious, emerge. I realised that for me these feelings or attitudes had been there for many years and that the story of Peter was just one variant of a long line of uncommon, but important incidents. More than that, I can recall each of these dilemmas, several of which caused me frustration or anger, and also a deep sense of personal failure, which I hid behind the criticism of others. Ironically I often preach that to do palliative care well one has to be generous. Being generous to the patients and families is relatively easy. Being generous to one's colleague is more difficult and being generous to oneself harder still. As soon as I began to think in this vein I started to make progress. First I looked back to my own days in general practice and tried to put myself in the position of my GP colleague in this incident and to understand, and more important, to feel how he felt. This is what I experienced by standing in his shoes.

He was a member of an excellent and well respected practice with high ideals. He accepted absolutely that high technical expertise in medicine should be sought from specialists and that one should not be too proud, but refer rapidly as soon as the situation warranted it. However, palliative care was a vital part of the GP's role and having a good team around him he was keen, as they were, to do it well.

As things progressed with Peter the GP tried harder and harder, perhaps becoming aware that daily or twice daily visits were a bit 'over the top'. But because Peter's problems were proving tricky, he had little option. As the community nurses became involved, the practice developed a mini-support team for Peter to deal with these issues. However, things continued to go less well than usual and certainly not as he would have liked them to do.

To return one weekend and find that the family had spoken to a medical friend, who in turn had spoken to the palliative care consultant for his advice, impugned his professional ability and made him defensive. He was also justly critical of the ethics of what the consultant had done. At this point his efforts re-doubled and some weeks later it was a great relief to go on holiday and perhaps an even greater relief to return to find that Peter had died while he had been away. The involvement of the palliative care specialist was then an irrelevancy. He might even have taken the view that although he had not needed it, understandably, his younger, less experienced partner did. But now he could support Margaret in her bereavement and give her all the care she requested.

As soon as I, the writer, looked at the GP's dilemma in this way I was able to identify with his feelings and to recognise what I knew as commonplace amongst all doctors, myself included, wherever they work and practice. I must recognise that although I do not feel a threat to others, that is not how others see me. I also have to realise that I have a reputation, which exists, for good or ill, and that people will talk about me, well or badly as the case may be.

Although I have never met the doctor concerned, he must in some way see me as a threat. This reminds me of Lord Hill's comment about how ability and expertise should be hidden by a relaxed and benign exterior if any personal success is to be achieved. Despite his high intellect and great ability, Lord Hill hid behind the bumbling image of the radio doctor of the Second World War, with enormous success.

Theory in use: the way ahead

So how should I use this incident constructively and for the benefit of patients and families, other health care professionals and for palliative care in today's NHS? Also how could I use it for myself? I decided to take the advice of a senior civil servant, who once told me that in his metaphorical hip pocket, he carried twenty things which he would like to achieve in order of priority. He had long since learned that one cannot begin at the beginning and go through the list in turn from one to twenty because the *political or other climate will not be right.* In his wisdom, he took an opportunist stance. When the Minister expressed a sudden interest in a particular issue, say care in the community, and it was one of the items on his list, he would take advantage of this to move that issue forward. Whether it was the first item or the last on his list was irrelevant. The *political climate was now right* for this particular issue, so it immediately became top priority. Without the list, opportunities would not arise with the same force. With the list his patience was rewarded and the department could focus on a clear, achievable goal now that it had political support.

This enabled him to avoid impossible or exhausting battles and to focus the department's skills on what the Minister had now made a real possibility.

I too had to formulate a new theory:

1 That I had to be more generous with my colleagues, especially those with whom it was not easy to be generous. I had no idea of the background of the people involved and how or why they found it easy or difficult to seek help from colleagues. Instead of being critical (which was about me), I needed to be less of a threat and more empathetic, understanding and constructive.
2 That the management of Peter was infinitely better than it would have been twenty years ago and that this was a reason for celebration: a strength on which further improvement could be built.
3 The competitive nature of today's health service is not in the interest of patients. We, the practitioners of whatever discipline, must collaborate, work together and complement each other's skills.
4 This can only be achieved by better dialogue in future and the development of opportunities for *learning* on both sides.

Having worked my way through these thoughts, the opportunity I was seeking unexpectedly occurred. My department was approached by senior general practitioners and community nurses, who, speaking on behalf of their colleagues, wished to develop their skills in palliative care in order that their patients would benefit and their teams would feel greater satisfaction and less stress. As a result collaborative meetings are under way in which I am learning to listen, to be generous and to support our colleagues in developing real ownership of the project without fear of being 'taken over'. I am elated. I look pleased and that in itself makes others feel optimistic and supported. For my part, I find the whole prospect exciting, but the particular pay off and satisfaction to me will be watching the inevitable enjoyment my colleagues experience and the closer relationship with them, which will inevitably occur.

Conclusion

Following this incident and my penultimate thoughts about the way ahead, I was invited to speak at a conference on how I coped with personal crises in medicine. The essence of the conference was to explore what health professionals and professionals in other settings do when there is absolutely nothing else left to do. As I planned my lecture, attended the conference, learned from others and re-wrote my talk twenty-four hours before I gave it, I realised how opportune all this had been. The Peter story, the construction and thought behind this chapter, our collaboration with GPs and the conference itself, all brought together dilemmas which I had half consciously and half unconsciously struggled with for over twenty years. I began to find solutions to issues I had found difficult and to feel a metaphorical weight fall from my shoulders generating a relief and freedom in professional work which I had not felt for years. This is the epitome of reflection in practice. So to return to those people who are 'doing reflective practice all the time', I have sympathy. This one incident has involved not only my professional practice, but my thoughts, attitudes and feelings built up over a lifetime.

It has been hard physical and emotional work. Though exhausting, it has been an exciting and stimulating and, I hope, a fruitful journey, but I do not think I could indulge in reflective practice all the time; maybe in another twenty years.

Chapter 8

Supporting students in undergraduate research: anxieties, ambiguities and agendas

Sheila Reading

Background

As a nurse teacher one of my areas of responsibility includes co-ordinating and teaching on a research skills module for qualified nurses, midwives and health visitors who are registered for a part time degree. The module, which currently extends over eighteen months, enables students to explore research both in relation to their own area of practice and in the wider context of health care provision. During the module students are required to undertake a practice-based research project with academic supervision. The students are generally experienced practitioners, many of whom are in senior roles. Many encounter a range of conflicts when returning to adult education on a part time basis while continuing to carry the usual work responsibilities.

Having gained several years' experience in this particular role, constantly monitoring and evaluating various aspects relating to the module, I feel I have quite a reasonable appreciation of the main issues associated with it. Yet there are some situations which tend to keep reappearing and find me struggling to understand and appreciate what is happening and why. I find great difficulty tackling these practice problems and recognise that I fail to resolve them. Perhaps that is because I remember the uncomfortable feelings about the problem but do not critically analyse the implications for practice. However I recently decided to confront one of these incidents in order to understand it better and with the aim of understanding and improving my professional actions and behaviour.

The critical incident

At the end of a group tutorial one morning I was speaking informally to a few students, hoping to gauge how work on their research projects was progressing. The projects were due to be completed during the next month and I knew most of the students were working closely with their research supervisor and were near to completion. As I listened to the conversations of their experiences it was clear that some students were grappling with the usual difficulties of writing up a research dissertation, but at the same time were making satisfactory progress and saw an end to the task in sight. Looking at my watch I reminded myself that I needed to leave the group and go to my next lecture. I picked up my files and prepared to leave the room. In doing so I made eye contact with Mary, one of the more quiet members of the group. Stopping briefly I asked her how she was getting on with writing up her report. This question resulted in Mary pouring out her problems. She replied that she was not having much success with writing. Her supervisor had been away for a few weeks and Mary had found she was unable to write anything about the research method she was using. She suggested that she did not really understand it once she had come to write about it, even though she had managed to collect her data. Mary had used an action research approach to develop and improve an aspect of her clinical practice.

Initial thoughts and feelings

I found myself trying to understand how Mary had collected data using a method she did not understand. Why, I wondered, had this only become apparent at this late stage. Would she have time to complete writing up the research project? Did she even understand what she had researched?

I was regretting having stopped to ask her this question as I had not really been prepared for this reply. I could feel myself listening to her but not wanting to hear what she was saying. I began to panic as all sorts of thoughts came into my head at once. I struggled to make sense out of what was being said by the student, at the same time thinking "I do not believe this. Does she really mean she has carried out a research project and collected data without understanding the method? How can she have got to this stage and not mentioned this to me? Has she told her supervisor this? Has she been meeting with her supervisor? How can she be at this point in the module and so close to presenting her written project without understanding the method used in her research study and why? Has the module failed in some way to make her aware of her responsibilities, and have I as the module co-ordinator got to accept some blame? Are other students in this predicament?"

In attempting to make sense of what I was hearing, I became anxious for Mary. Her research dissertation was due for assessment very shortly and I could relate to her stress – failure was always a possibility. Mary was a student who had had difficulties on previous occasions in articulating her ideas verbally and in writing. I sensed her concern about this but struggled now about how I might help her at this time.

What to do?

As I was expected at another lecture there was no time to stop and deal adequately with this. Furthermore, even as I struggled to think when I might be available to meet with her and talk the situation through, I remembered I was not going to be at the School again until early the following week. I was in turmoil. Having invited the student to reveal this information to me, I felt obliged to respond and yet at the same time I was thinking that she could not expect me to abandon all my commitments and resolve the situation there and then. I tried to view things from the student's perspective – having been asked about her progress, she had felt able to indicate that she had a problem and her supervisor was not available to help her. As the module co-ordinator I was in a position to offer support, or at least she might have had expectations that I should address the problem. Interestingly Mary had not asked explicitly for any assistance, this was my interpretation of the situation. I was now feeling very uncomfortable. I was agitated too that I needed to leave then if I were to keep my next appointment and at the same time needed to resolve this dilemma decisively and quickly.

The situation was making me feel angry, both with myself and with the student. Why had I stopped to speak to her and why had she responded to a polite, routine enquiry in such a way? Why was I upset that she had shared her problem with me? In the midst of all these thoughts and feelings I had to make some speedy decisions. On the one hand I considered she was an adult learner, the problem had not just occurred at that moment and there was little that I could do there and then. On the other hand 'something' had to be done to show I had acknowledged the problem and would respond as soon as I was able.

All this happened in the space of about a minute. I had listened to her, only speaking to clarify her situation. I was concerned that my reactions, verbal and non-verbal, were perhaps negative and aggressive because of my anxiety and annoyance. This was not the professional manner I would ever choose but my emotions pre-vented me from behaving as I would have preferred, that is calmly, clearly and with confidence. At last I spoke to tell her I was sorry to learn that she was having difficulties and explained I did not have time then – indeed not until the next week – to spend more time dealing with her situation. I advised her to meet with her supervisor as soon as possible to discuss the situation, and suggested she write a note to her supervisor immediately explaining the situation in detail and requesting an urgent appointment.

It was difficult for me to gauge how much insight the student had into her situation and whether she recognised the implications of what she had just suggested about her research project. Did she really not understand the research method, or was it just that she could not write about it? There was no time to stop and assess this now and that made me feel powerless to help. I hesitated again for a moment. A sudden insight made me recognise that I was taking control of the situation and directing her. This added to my feeling of discomfort. In an attempt to involve the student in resolving the situation, I asked her what she felt she could usefully do before meeting with her supervisor and whether she felt there was any-thing she thought I could do to help. She shook her head and explained that she felt she had already tried everything to overcome her problem and did not know what to do next. This was interpreted by me as her wanting something tangible from me. I responded by offering to send some articles and references which were relevant to the research method and then offered to meet with her as soon as I could the following week. Whether I did this to make her feel better or to help me feel better is questionable. The fact was that I then felt I could end the encounter. Summarising the main action plan I left the room – and the student.

As I walked down the corridor I became even more aware of how I was feeling. I was red faced and feeling very stressed. Now I had to rush somewhere else and turn up late, looking quite unprofessional! In addition I sensed I had totally mishandled the situation. I felt angry. As co-ordinator of the module I felt I was partly to blame that Mary was in this position. A 'good' module surely would prevent students having problems like this. On top of that it had not been possible to handle the situation as I would have liked – I had failed to solve the problem for her. The time constraint had been another thing to be angry about. There never seemed to be enough time to spend with students. Equally I recognised the need to help students to become independent and autonomous learners, able to confront and deal with uncertain and difficult situations. While students ultimately have to take responsibility for their learning, teachers have a role in facilitating that learning. That is one of my strongly upheld beliefs. Learning is not entirely a 'do it yourself' concern.

Reflecting – a change of tactics

I mulled over this incident for some time, sometimes feeling angry with the student and at other times feeling angry with 'the system'. Most of the time I was annoyed with myself and remained uncomfortable and disheartened about my professional practice during that incident. The temptation was to forget it and get on with life. There was no further time to be wasted on the matter. That was how I normally coped with a practice problem. Incidents such as this, when students seem to struggle with learning and where I am unable to clarify what the reasons for this are, leave me feeling helpless. The question I needed to ask was, why? On this occasion I decided to try to analyse the incident and write about it. In the process I could explore it in more detail, questioning my thoughts and reactions. I felt dissatisfied with what had happened and thought I could usefully explore some of the issues it presented me with in order to learn from my practice.

Turning to the literature on reflection I found many ideas which spoke to me about how I might explore my practice incident. In particular I identified with the idea of self-reflective enquiry undertaken by teachers wishing to improve their own social and educational practice and understand more about that practice and the institution and context within which it occurs (Kemmis, 1985, p. 156).

Attempting to make sense of the incident and my reactions

The early struggle

Schön (1983) proposes that the situations of practice are not problems to be solved, but instead are problematic situations where there exists uncertainty and disorder. I felt I was not necessarily searching for a solution but rather trying to understand why the incident had made me feel 'embroiled in conflicts of values, goals, purposes and interests' (Schön, 1983, p. 10). The many personal and professional and organisational conflicts of the encounter with Mary had bothered me and the incident had found me unable to behave or practise professionally in the way that I would wish.

As I grappled with the thoughts and feelings aroused by the incident, I recognised that there were many issues and questions embedded in this situation. They concerned such things as: what is my role as a lecturer in enabling students to be self-directing, autonomous adult learners; what is the purpose of a research dissertation for undergraduate practitioners; why was this student having difficulties with the research method and writing it up; why was I so uncomfortable with the situation?

The discomfort

Schön (1983) was right about the uncertainties – there were many in this practice incident. As I thought about some of them, I recognised that I was personally uncomfortable and unsure how to deal with them. I am the sort of person who prefers everything to be neat and tidy and to remain in control, personally and professionally. While I recognise that practice is by its very nature messy, I always consider my own practice is only messy when I have failed in some way! I struggled with the paradox presented to me as I reflected on this and saw that I could no longer ignore the gulf between what I believe about practice (in my head) and what I do in reality (in my actions and behaviour). It was challenging to see myself so clearly in this way; it allowed me to see how I behave in practice in a new light.

I could also see that as I had tried to make sense of Mary's situation, I had produced interpretations based on my own ideas and beliefs about learning and research. Those ideas initially suggested to me that if there was a problem then the student needed to work harder to solve it. After all, the other students seemed to be on top of the situation. It was as if I considered that only poor or lazy students experience difficulties. (It is the case though, that experience has shown me that it is the motivated and thinking students who question things.) These conflicts in my thinking were illuminating both personally and professionally. However, I was still faced with this uncertainty – was Mary not working hard enough, or was she experiencing particular difficulties in writing up her research? My knowledge of her suggested she did not spend much time reading and often refused to present her academic work because she had been too busy with clinical work.

I did not feel confident enough at the time of the incident to say to Mary that her struggle had great potential for her learning and understanding more about the whole process of research. Knowing the difficulties she had to contend with, being a part time student, I chose to believe that if she spent more time reading around the topic, writing drafts of her research method and communicating with her supervisor, the problems would resolve.

Why I thought in this way reveals much about myself and my practice. Within these lie my own complex values, beliefs and theories about the research process and adult professional learning. I was very surprised and challenged to discover the differences between what I thought I believed and what my actions reveal about my beliefs. At the same time it is exciting as I see the potential to alter how I respond and behave in future.

Agendas

Reflection enabled me to identify and examine several different agendas in undergraduate research. Mary had to produce a dissertation as evidence of having undertaken her own research study. While that process enabled her to learn research skills, she also needed to achieve a pass grade when assessed by internal and external assessors in order to graduate. She may have felt uncertain about her decision to adopt an action research approach and how that might influence her final grade. Certainly the writing up of her research would not follow the more dominant positivist and interpretative research paradigms usually presented by health care professionals. Nor should it. But would that be acceptable to assessors to whom she was unknown who might have definite views about what constituted 'good' research? Again I felt some responsibility as module co-ordinator since I considered that I always encouraged students to explore research methods which they considered appropriate to their research topic. But was this disadvantaging them at assessment? I am very aware that my colleagues who are assessors have a range of views which are different from my own and how this may influence marks awarded. Once again it revealed another level of my own uncertainty about the purpose of the research dissertation. I encouraged students to view it as a significant learning process; one in which they should learn from errors and mistakes. But it was also to be assessed as a product – warts and all.

As well as the assessment agenda, I was aware that Mary could have a different agenda about what she hoped to achieve from writing the research dissertation, in terms of learning, and how she might use it in practice. I had not taken time to explore her agenda(s) at the time of the incident. Anxiety had made me focus on my agendas and those of the organisation of which I am part.

Writing and reflecting

I needed to explore the practice incident from many different perspectives. Having written down the incident and my feelings I found further questions emerging about my behaviour and actions. How might the student have felt about the interaction? What would have made the incident seem more manageable for her and for me? What is there to learn from all this which can improve my professional practice?

As I read and re-read what I had written about the incident, words and phrases jumped out at me. Many of them startled and surprised me. It was clear that the action of writing about the practice incident had enabled me to see aspects of my practice which I had not been aware of before. I was shocked by some of the thoughts and feelings I had written down, and later wanted to disbelieve, even deny them. Surely I had not felt angry with the student ... was that possible? I was beginning to learn some things about myself that were uncomfortable. This was further painful evidence that aspects of my actual practice were incongruent with my desired practice. Argyris (1976) has indicated that espoused theories can be different from theories in use.

Knowing and learning from practice

Carper (1978) described four ways of knowing in nursing: the empirical, the personal, the ethical and the aesthetic. Using this framework to explore the practice incident I saw that there were gaps in all these ways of knowing about my practice. Or, perhaps to put it another way, there were four ways of *not* knowing revealed in the practice incident. There were aspects of 'self' which I had not recognised, or chosen not to recognise, in my professional actions (personal knowing). In addition there was a dissonance between what I believed I was, an adult educator who tried to be student focused and work to establish good teacher–student relationships, and what I actually felt and did in practice. Examining the art of my practice (examining the experienced whole in order to perceive what is there, Carper, 1978, p. 17), has revealed a gap in my knowing. Ethical knowing is to do with making decisions about the right thing to do in practice. I had certainly struggled at the time not knowing how to do the best thing for the student. I considered that perhaps I did not have to hand the theoretical knowledge (empirical knowledge) needed in that situation to make the 'right' professional judgement for the situation.

The question was: what was the required theoretical knowledge? Formal theories about research and adult learning have their place but the incident highlighted the complexity and uncertainty of professional practice. Formal theories are not always helpful in guiding one through the uncertainties of practice. Here I tend to rely on past experience and intuition – personal theories. So often I have joked with colleagues about a situation that 'they' did not teach us about at university. Yet in this incident and the ensuing reflection my personal theories were being scrutinised and I saw the need to change them. In practice and in reality there are no absolute truths or certainties to hold on to. Practice occurs in an ever-changing culture and context. I am very aware of the change in nurse education during the last decade and the accompanying need for practitioners to develop research skills for practice.

Recognising the need to learn more about the incident, I felt a need to review some literature and formal theories relevant to my practice. This revealed my more common approach to learning – using theory to direct my practice. I later recognised the conflicts which that produced for me.

Adult education and the self-directed learner

Knowles (1990) believed adult learners are ready to learn and are self-directing. However, it may actually be threatening for learners to be self-directed if in the past they have always been directed by others. Recognising this, Jarvis (1983) indicates that some students may require considerable support and assistance from teachers to become self-directing and independent. But I am not sure to what extent I truly encourage students to be self-directing, or whether in some way I inhibit their independence. Clearly there are implications here for how I work with students to encourage them to learn from the uncertainties of the research process. Perhaps I could have been more positive about Mary's situation and should have encouraged her to see the challenges that existed within her uncertainties. Nevertheless there is also a need to get the right balance between too little and too much support (Brown, 1993).

Davies (1976) argues that rather than being student centred, the curriculum should be enquiry centred with a focus on the process of learning. The student then would not have a 'freedom to learn' (Rogers, 1983) but a responsibility to learn. This may be worth exploring further in the current climate of education in the 1990s.

As a teacher I still struggle with having to accept that there may come a point when students fail to pass a course module. I need to develop my confidence and skills in order to recognise where my responsibilities end and where student learning begins. In the meantime I could be more active in incorporating strategies that can help students become student centred learners. Grow (1991) suggests that it may be necessary to 'model' or demonstrate the skills of self-directed learning. Clearly I need to deal with the ambiguities in my own practice before I can be in a position to model skills. In analysing this incident I became aware of the fact I may be communicating one message verbally while communicating the opposite in my actions. 'Do as I say, not what I do' is not the appropriate model for an adult educator.

Knowles (1990) focuses on the importance of the individual learner in the learning process, the individual's experience and the learner's perception of relevance. Here was the direction for me to refocus my practice. During the incident I focused mainly on my own personal feelings and professional interpretations rather than understanding Mary's perspective. Perhaps that was as a result of personal stress.

Stress

I recognised that the constraints of the real world of education in which I function often generate stress. This caused me to focus on those aspects of my role over which I can exert control. Looking instead at the student and how I could facilitate her learning and understanding of research would be a much more appropriate approach. The lack of a student focus may be a defence against anxiety (Menzies, 1970). Benner (1984) also suggests that stress derives from a context where there is a lack of resources and little to empower the individual. Too often I am conscious of a lack of time for interacting with students in the ways I would like. This and other constraints of the job serve to disempower me and lead to a sense of dissatisfaction. Nor do I doubt that students also feel disempowered.

The anger I felt during the encounter with Mary was caused by the conflicts which I experienced in the practice incident. It would be all too easy to blame the student. Yet the anger derived from the complexity of practice. I recognised that I was angry for many reasons. Reflecting on this, I consider the anger was to do with all the turmoil I was experiencing during the incident. Initially I felt angry with the student, then I turned it on myself and then was angry with the 'system' within which I have to operate. I recognised the anger as a symptom of stress.

With further time to reflect I see there are implications here for personal, professional and curriculum changes. After all, the 'system' which I externalise is what I am part of. As I change and develop my practice I can influence the curriculum and resources needed.

Context

As I analysed and reflected longer on these issues I saw the incident in a broader perspective. The issues were not just about adult education but also about the arena in which it takes place. Discussions about the purpose of research education, what methods are justifiable, the process and outcomes of research dissertations, all occur within a particular context. Schools of Nursing and Midwifery are designed to fulfil certain social and professional functions. While they operate within the arena of Higher Education and reflect the needs of the National Health Service, I also recognise that these organisations exist within the wider social and cultural environment of the 1990s. In focusing on the broader context, however, it is easy too to overlook the student's personal agenda and to forget the context within which she comes to be on the course, her motives, stresses and needs. Both contexts need to be borne in mind.

Conflict and nurse education

I am certain that the conflict of values which I experienced between theories in use and espoused theories is to some extent a reflection of the context within which I work as a teacher. The curriculum makes philosophical beliefs explicit. That is, the learner is autonomous and accepts responsibility for her own learning. The teacher is a facilitator of learning. The function of education is continuing development of the professional. Yet as Hendricks-

Thomas and Patterson (1995) point out, an overt curriculum espousing critical thinking and humanism co-exists with a covert curriculum directed by a means–ends rationality. Ironically it is an assessment-driven curriculum which dictates the shape of nurse education today as it takes its place within the university setting.

That is not to say things cannot be changed but rather to appreciate the constraints that currently exist. There was, in the incident described, a need to ensure that this student would complete the research project, and the module, which competed with the need to help the student become more questioning of research ambiguities and more confident about her own judgements and abilities. Abercrombie, cited by Nias (1995), argues that students and teachers encourage authority dependence, albeit unconsciously, and the result of this is that students have problems in making independent judgements, have reduced capacity to use new information productively and are inhibited in their creativity. I am certain this is how I colluded with Mary on this occasion. Conscious of this, I shall try to remain aware of it in the future. Acknowledging the context in which I work and in which I continually feel that I am required to 'do' more, I should also question whether I should instead try to 'be' more for the student (Shannon, 1991).

The students' perspective

Adult learners need help to become self-directed (Jarvis, 1983). Mary, like many experienced nurses, was encountering an education system which has changed considerably in the last decade. It is likely that her previous experience as a student nurse had not prepared her for the uncertainties of undergraduate education. While she had a wealth of personal and professional experience she possibly lacked confidence in her academic ability. My knowledge of her made me believe that she did not have high expectations of herself. Often students like Mary have not had an opportunity to develop those skills required to organise, plan and present their work.

While some attention is given to this by teachers, students are expected to be able to be self-directing and develop these skills through negotiation with teaching and other academic staff. There may be difficulties for some individuals in achieving this at an appropriate stage of their learning, particularly if they are unwilling to admit their problems or (which is even worse) are not aware of them. It is possible that Mary was faced with this predicament as her assessment deadline approached. She may have been seeking help in a manner with which she has become familiar in an earlier educational experience. How did she feel about my response? This I can only guess at, but believe she was dismayed that I did not adopt a more nurturing and supporting role.

In considering why I did not do more for her I recognise the personal and organisational constraints influencing me at that time. In addition I am aware of the conflict I was experiencing between wanting to treat her as an autonomous adult learner and wanting to take control of her dilemma and sort it all out for her there and then. The constraints of the situation and the context of adult education forced the issue for me, but I was uncomfortable, both personally and professionally, and as a result offered to follow her up as soon as I could and provide some references in the meantime. The compromise was uncomfortable and I felt unsure of the ethics of the situation. What would have been the right thing to do? The question is: right for whom, and why? Clearly the answer to this lies at the heart of my learning from the incident.

Professional beliefs and values

My views about adult learning and my values, attitudes and beliefs have evolved during my professional and personal life. Professional behaviour is determined to some extent by the current organisational context but also by a life history and experiences. I am aware that my upbringing encouraged me to do things to the best of my abilities and that a strong work ethic pervades all areas of my life. I seem to abide by an old adage which I recall hearing my grandmother frequently repeat during my childhood, 'if a job is worth doing, it is worth doing well'. I accepted personal responsibility from an early age for the outcomes of my learning experiences. Success or failure I believe lie within my control.

It seemed as though I treated Mary as if she had the same control over her destiny. Considering this carefully I saw that attitude made me redundant as a facilitator and module co-ordinator. The practice incident was revealing further conflicts between what I claimed to believe and what I experienced. Indeed as I consider the idea of control, I recognise that none of us has complete control over every situation. The incident had made me uncomfortable because I could not control it as I wanted. Somehow my professional practice needed to reflect that knowing.

The incident also highlighted the issue of my need to care and help others – perhaps why I became a nurse. These caring values, which I still espouse as a nurse teacher, may need to be reassessed. In the case of this practice incident involving Mary I was aware of some incongruence in my feelings. In part I wanted her to recognise the strengths of acknowledging uncertainties, but my caring values caused me to want to do something practical to help her. I may need now to consider how 'care' differs in the educational environment from the clinical environment and clarify these differences for myself.

Focusing on lessons from practice

I was beginning to be overwhelmed by my analysis of my practice. In exploring the incident there was so much learning happening but where was it all leading? I was doubting the value of continuing to explore the literature, indeed I was getting a little bored with it. I 'knew' all these things already. I had spent time studying it; it just seemed that in practice it was not that simple to apply. Why was this?

At that time I read an article given to me by a colleague who knew I was engaged in some reflective writing. This article was different from anything else I had read on reflection – why? Suddenly I knew the reason. It was not an exposition about the potential or scope of reflection, nor about how to reflect on practice. It was instead a practitioner's own written reflective account of practice (Landgrebe and Winter, 1994). The writing took the form of two stories, both of which moved me to tears. Each powerfully illustrated, without recourse to formal or theoretical references, how practitioners learn from their own practice. The theory in these instances emerged from practice.

I decided to set aside all the texts and articles sprawled around my desk and to look afresh at the practice incident. After all, I bring to my practice many years of experience in education and life. In that recognition I gained a new perspective. Exploring again the incident involving Mary, I suddenly saw her perspective more clearly. It seemed that my struggle to reflect analytically about my practice was not dissimilar to her struggle to write up her research dissertation. I too had come to a point when I was unsure about what I was doing and lacked confidence in my own abilities. At that point I had turned to the literature to search for the formal theories which might help me. But they could not – theoretical knowledge is only one aspect of practice and on its own it is quite useless. How true were Landgrebe and Winter's words: 'No amount of theoretical knowledge can prepare any practitioner to cope with the variety of situations and events with which he/she will be presented' (1994, p. 89).

Perhaps Mary had found that all the theory about how to write up her research method did not help her in practice. As a teacher it was for me to support and help her with this task. Instead I had focused on why the problem had happened and how I could prevent it happening again. Neither of these two issues were of immediate concern and only served to divert my attention from the problem at hand. I only needed to deal with Mary's present problem. There would be time later to analyse it and learn the lessons for the future.

It seemed the other lesson that the incident was teaching me was that I needed to accept that problems will always arise. Perfect as I would like things to be, I operate in the real world. Instead I should expect and accept problems in practice. Through this acceptance I could see further possibilities. Not only was it possible that I would cope better with problems, but that they would actually become the occasions when I could analyse and further develop my professional practice. Perhaps I too could learn to be less stressed by difficulties and uncertainties experienced in practice.

New confidence in practice

I have learned so much through reflecting on, writing about and talking with peers about this one practice incident. Some of it has been painful and some exciting. Not least I have discovered a new way to develop and improve my practice. But beyond the insight and learning about my educational practice I have experienced something else – a new confidence. When I embarked on writing this chapter I had little to guide me other than an assurance from others that there was no right or wrong way to do it – just my way. In the process I have evolved my own style. It strikes me that is how each of us practises (with our own distinctive style) and yet it is embedded within a tradition of practice. While we may all practise differently there are common approaches, and by exploring individual practices we can each learn something new.

Conclusions – but not the end

The outcomes of this exploration of an aspect of my practice have indeed been unexpected (Boud, Keogh and Walker, 1985). However, the purpose of the investigation of practice was to discover an understanding of it, of myself and the context within which I practise. It was not a process intended to make me more aware of inadequacies, my own or those of the 'system'. Indeed it was to gain encouragement rather than to be discouraged that I undertook this enquiry into a difficult incident. I started out with the hope of developing my practice and have gained insights which have undoubtedly developed me personally as well as professionally. The focus of my practice has altered during the process of critically examining it. This has been a new way of looking at my practice. It has taught me to focus on the student and the context within which he or she is functioning. It is too easy when one is stressed to become focused on your own thoughts and feelings.

It has reminded me too how quickly we adapt to situations and accept certain happenings without stopping to learn from them, and how quickly practice becomes 'routine' and we lose sight of what is influencing our professional actions and interventions. But knowing something in theory is not the same as knowing it in practice, or even doing it in practice. A lot of things will get in the way of my practice ever being perfect but an appreciation of the complexities helps me to cope.

To develop my professional practice requires a commitment. Too often in the 'busy-ness' of daily practice I have failed to return to those uncomfortable experiences which could perhaps help me most to develop. There is always more to continue thinking about

– and so my professional practice will continue to grow and develop – and in a constantly changing context – the process will never end. Nor indeed has the learning from this single practice incident really ended.

References

Argyris, C. (1976). Theories of action that inhibit individual learning. *American Psychologist,* 1, 638–654.

Benner, P. (1984). *From Novice to Expert: Excellence and Power in Clinical Nursing Practice.* Addison-Wesley.

Boud, D., Keogh, R. and Walker, D. (eds.) (1985). *Reflection: Turning Experience into Learning.* Kogan Page.

Brown, G. D. (1993). Accounting for power: nurse teachers' and students' perceptions of power in their relationships. *Nurse Education Today,* 13, 111–120.

Carper, B. A. (1978). Fundamental patterns of knowing in nursing. *Advances in Nursing Science,* 1, 13–23.

Davies, I. K. (1976). *Objectives in Curriculum Design.* McGraw-Hill.

Grow, A. (1991). Teaching learners to be self directed. *Adult Education Quarterly ,* 41, 125–129.

Hendricks-Thomas, J. and Patterson, E. (1995). A sharing in critical thought by nursing faculty. *Journal of Advanced Nursing,* 22, 594–599.

Jarvis, P. (1983). *Professional Education.* Croom Helm.

Kemmis, S. (1985). Action research and the politics of reflection. In *Reflection: Turning Experience into Learning* (D. Boud, R. Keogh and D. Walker, eds.), pp. 139–164. Kogan Page.

Knowles, M. (1990). *The Adult Learner: A Neglected Species.* (4th Edn). Gulf Publishers.

Landgrebe, B. and Winter, R. (1994). 'Reflective' writing on practice: professional support for the dying? *Educational Action Research,* 2, 83–94.

Menzies, I. (1970). *The Functioning of Social Systems as a Defence against Anxiety.* Pamphlet No. 5, Tavistock.

Nias, J. (1995). Developing intellectual independence. *New Academic,* 4, 8–9.

Rogers, C. R. (1983). *Freedom to Learn for the 80s.* Charles E. Merrill.

Schön, D. A. (1983). *The Reflective Practitioner: How Professionals Think in Action.* Basic Books.

Shannon, A. (1991). The future of nursing. *Nursing,* 4, 26–28.

Chapter 9

Agonising about assessment

Judith Chapman

Introduction

I have been assessing physiotherapy students for more than twenty years. Despite an inescapable underlying tension around assessment, I have noticed that some colleagues appear quite comfortable and confident when considering a student's professional abilities in an assessment context. Doubt and uncertainty, however, frequently accompany me when I assess academic or clinical performances. I constantly struggle to assure myself that I can discriminate correctly between students, and that I can justify the marks I award. This personal altercation has stimulated a long term interest in assessment instruments and procedures that foster accuracy and reproducibility when marking.

In this chapter, I shall describe several events that pertain to assessing physiotherapy students, both in the clinical field and in the academic environment. These events led up to a recent critical incident, which shifted and changed my thinking and outlook on assessments. I will discuss the events that occurred, relating them to a theoretical basis for assessment.

When I was first asked to write this chapter, I immediately put myself into the role of 'the expert'. I expected to explore the subject and come up with definitive answers for you, the reader. As I engaged in the subject, my anxiety reached an all time high because I was not coming up with answers. I read more and more. Each author convinced me that his or her approach to assessment was the 'right' answer. But, since each approach was different and based on different educational paradigms, I could not sort out which was the best. Even if I could choose, would the approach(es) be useful to you in your environment? What I have done then, in writing this chapter, is to present several situations that were memorable to me in my career as an educator. It is not so much the answers that I came up with that I wish you to take away with you. Rather, I hope to illustrate the process of reflection in such a way that you can use it to critique your own unique experiences and make your own discoveries and decisions about your approach to assessments and what will work for you.

Insight (1)

When I was planning my writing for this chapter, I expected to describe the most recent critical event and reflect on the feelings and the issues that it uncovered (Schön, 1987). I expected to generate questions and follow through with a theoretical exploration of the ideas (Boud *et al.*, 1993). I expected to conclude with how the exercise had altered the way I dealt with assessments. I found, however, that as I started to write, my thoughts kept returning to other critical events that had shaped my response to the latest event. I was still confused about the meaning of the critical event, and certainly, at that time, did not know how to look for any answers. I was still feeling defensive about events that had taken place and was looking to justify the decisions and actions that I had taken. I could not allow myself to be open to new ideas that could evolve from the situation. In fact, now that I think about it, I had been stuck for six months plus, resisting looking closely at the recommendations made to me at that time. I therefore decided to leave the event and record those important incidents that I felt led me to be where I was with my thinking and actions at the time of the critical event. Postel (1993) emphasises the need to 'attend to the whole of our experience', indicating the importance of discovering the influences of past experiences on current behaviour. Perhaps my history with assessments is so much an integral part of the foundation for my future learning that I need to explore the preceding events that led to the critical incident in order to understand it fully.

Post Script

The process that I have been through in writing this chapter, and the conclusions I've drawn, certainly support the formal theory espoused by Postel. In tracing my evolving understanding of assessment over time, I have managed to uncover some of my personal driving forces that influence the way I carry out assessments on students (subjectivity), which up until now I have tried to ignore or bury in my search for flawless objectivity.

For me to be able to write this chapter, I had to approach the critical events that led up to the incident in a chronological order. Partly, as I have explained, it related to my inability to get in touch with the feelings triggered by the event. Recently, however, I have uncovered two other reasons for this approach.

One is that if I show you how I have developed my competency as an examiner, you might not judge my 'failure' so harshly. Having read about the events leading up to it you will understand the context in which I was operating.

The other is that the assessment of professional skills has changed dramatically over the past twenty years. I have been involved with those changes and wanted to share the progression of thoughts over time so that you can more easily understand the complexity of the situation that faced me at the culmination of events.

If, however, you feel that you can gain more by reading about the critical incident first, please go to page 172 and then revert to this part of the text and fit the information into the context of the understanding you had when exploring the critical incident.

I am also aware that inserting my insights into the text, as I go along, may interfere with the train of thought you would develop as the descriptive events unfold. The material is presented for your learning, so approach it in whichever way stimulates your understanding and insight.

The events leading to the critical incident

How are educators trained to assess?

Race (1995), in his article on 'The Art of Assessing', states that lecturers in Higher Education are expected to teach and to assess students. He points out that, whereas there is often training for new staff who have had no formal instruction in *teaching*, few lecturers spend time learning about or practising how to *assess* students, except when 'on the job'. Because there is often little discussion about assessment and very little feedback on how well you do it (except from the odd irate or distressed student), assessing students can be a very nerve-wracking experience. It carries an enormous responsibility, because the assessor is making decisions that affect the student's career, and self-esteem in vocational education. He or she is also policing the standards for competent and safe practice, so the responsibility for assessment extends to the general public. How then, without proper training, does a lecturer develop competence in this activity? Physiotherapy educators used to have formal training in educational principles and practice (Turnbull, 1994), but, since the move into university-based programmes, this is no longer a prerequisite. There is more emphasis on the ability to engage in scholarly activities. So, even though educated to a masters or doctoral level, lecturers are often left with a serendipitous understanding of the learning process and assessment issues. Maybe because of the complex issues surrounding assessment, 'training' a lecturer is anyway inappropriate. Perhaps learning how to assess is a bit like parenting; you do it on the basis of your own experiences with it. If, however, you are educating and evaluating health professionals, a critical exploration of those experiences is imperative. The practice of reflection 'in' and 'on' action can be used to gain a greater understanding of, and more effective skills in, assessing student performance (Fish, 1989). So, as one (in)experienced educator to another, here goes!

Post Script

In reviewing my story, I can see that although I attended workshops on assessment and read the latest literature, the dilemmas I faced were never fully resolved. I leapt from one formal theory or model of practice to another trying to find answers to the fairest, most accurate way of assessing students. Each approach only answered part of the question. What I kept ignoring was my own *personal theory* about assessing. Unless I explore the internal influences and put them into the equation I will never get a full answer to the problem. The process of reflection that I have experienced in writing this chapter has influenced the way I assess students more significantly than any formal theory ever has.

My experience of assessments in the school system

Like most people, throughout school and my physiotherapy training I was tested constantly and assessments were a way of life. I trusted the assessment system and never questioned the examiners' ability to assess. If I did badly or well, it merely reflected how able I was in that particular subject. I relied implicitly on a fair judgement to be made by the assessor, and they would tell me the truth about my ability. Occasionally it occurred to me (or more truthfully, I hoped!) that the only reason I did not do well on something was because the teacher did not like me, but then I would think that the examiner knew what he or she was doing and that there were standards against which I was being assessed. It did cross my mind, especially when the assessment loomed in front of me, that I really had no idea what those standards were. I never actually knew what the examiner wanted of me bar memorising and regurgitating work that I had listened to in lectures or read out of a book. Presumably, the more I memorised the more likely I was to do well in the exam. Oh dear, why didn't I have a better memory? These feelings though seemed to differ according to the subject in which I was being examined. Maths for instance was straightforward. I was either right or wrong in my answers and it was easy to work out why. However, in English essays, history compositions, religious studies and dissertations it was more or less impossible to know what would get me a good mark. It seemed that even if I did memorise the content covered, I did not necessarily do well. I never figured out the more abstract qualities I needed in order to succeed. None of the teachers appeared able to explain them to me either. Somehow, it seemed to come from practice. In these situations the assessment and subsequent mark seemed to relate to the mood of the teacher at the time of marking and what his or her biases were. It appeared to me that for those topics where I could not memorise the material, either I had the ability or I did not. There was nothing more nor less that I could do about it. Such is the ignorance of the teenage years!

Insight (2)

There are indeed some subjects where the answers are clear cut, binomial; correct or incorrect; right or wrong. There may be aspects of some subjects in health professional education that are more amenable to 'objective' marking because they are more technical and observable. Then there are subjects or aspects of a subject that are more abstract. These concepts are not as readily defined or articulated and are consequently not free to be measured against specific criteria. It is difficult in these situations for an examiner to indicate exactly what influenced his or her judgement of the work or justify the mark given to the student. Hence, there is an element of 'subjectivity' in assessments, especially if what is being evaluated is the more abstract, higher order qualities (Bloom, 1974) of professional performance.

As educators of health professionals, we strive to develop the students' critical thinking skills and other complex characteristics that make up our professional practice (see Shepard and Jensen, 1990; Fish, 1991; Higgs, 1992a, 1992b; Fish, 1996). If they are difficult to define, how then do educators identify and assess these abstract qualities and convey to students what is expected of them? Professional practice is comprised of both observable actions or behaviours and professional attributes that are implicitly related to that performance. Do we then emphasise the assessment of the technical skills because these can be easily defined and marked, or should we explore the abstract issues more closely in an attempt to make them explicit for the benefit of the educator who is marking, as well as the student? Will this analysis of the elusive concepts reduce it to parts, which, when measured and aggregated again, would not reconstitute the whole we were attempting to assess (see Norman *et al.*, 1991)?

The tale unfolds

Assessing students in a clinical setting

I had only supervised one student's clinical placement when I was offered the opportunity to be a Clinical Instructor at McMaster University Medical Centre. This gave me the chance to move into a formal education environment. I was thrilled and accepted the challenges with enthusiasm. Most of the placement activities passed uneventfully, but I did find it difficult to monitor and facilitate the therapists' assessment of the students against a defined set of standards on the school's assessment form. I had had so little experience in the past with assessing students that I was unsure of how to acquire the ability to make those judgements. The standards given to us by the school were ambiguous and open to individual interpretation and I often found myself making different judgements about a student's performance from the therapist. I would attempt to guide therapists (with their inherent values, biases and differing levels of clinical competence) to interpret the standards in a consistent and identical manner. The sense of responsibility was onerous, for we had to judge the students' safety to practise, yet we could also destroy a student's career. I felt as though I was playing Russian Roulette. How would I get it right? Even if the therapists and I came to a mutual agreement, the students would often appeal against the mark, challenging us to be more specific about how the mark had been acquired and arguing that, because of the subjectivity of the therapist's judgement, in another department they would have been marked more leniently. (They never did query being marked more generously than in other departments!) I often wondered how long I could survive in this uncertainty, facing all these assessment dilemmas, without being discovered as a fraud (appearing as an expert, yet having no explicit or sound basis for my judgements).

To lessen my anxiety, I introduced an extension to the assessment system which would clarify the expectations between therapists and students. Students now set learning objectives, based on the school's assessment form, which specified outcome performances (skills, professional attitudes, knowledge base) that they would demonstrate in order to achieve their grades (Mager, 1975). When the assessment occurred, the student was much more aware of how successful (or not) he or she had been on the placement, because he or she was working on and evaluating clearly specified performances. All the time I was working on the notion that if students knew what was expected of them, then they would be more likely to achieve it. Also, setting objectives encouraged students to be active participants, and take responsibility for their own learning, which was an increasingly important underpinning of physiotherapy education and an integral part of Knowles' (1975) model of adult learning.

Insight (3)

Because I had not had any formal training in assessing students I fell back on my own experiences with school examinations to modify the students' clinical assessments. I was working on the assumption that the problem with assessments was that students did not clearly understand what was expected of them. If they did, they could work towards it at their own speed and in their own learning style and achieve. I assumed that given well-defined, negotiated objectives, and time, students could master any of the clinical challenges facing them. It would be a success story. No-one need fail.

I also assumed that any part of a clinical performance could be broken into definable, measurable, achievable tasks that could be observed and measured objectively. The tensions would be taken out of the assessment process.

Post Script

Throughout my six years as clinical instructor I struggled to get the clinical assessments as objective as possible. All the academic exams I had taken were 'objective'. What I had not realised then or articulated until recently was that it is more difficult to be clear about what is assessed (priorities) and the criteria used for judging clinical performance (weighting) in a one-to-one supervisor–student situation. Often, the relationship that builds up over the placement influences a therapist's ability to remain 'objective'. Ideas such as the following may affect their decisions.

- How much of the student's ultimate performance is dependent on the supervision received over the placement? To what extent will the final mark obtained by the student actually reflect how good the therapist is as a teacher?
- If the therapist likes the student and gets on well, is it more difficult to separate the person from the performance and give that student a lower mark than it is to give one to a student with whom there is little or no rapport, or even a 'personality clash'?
- In the absence of clear criteria an assessor often makes judgements on a student's performance, comparing one with another – (a little bit better than X, or a little bit worse than Y), eventually arriving at a spectrum of 'normal' against which he or

she can then judge a performance confidently. In the clinical setting, the therapists see only a few students in a year and it takes a long time to build up a repertoire of what is normal performance for a particular level of schooling. In the academic environment, where there are much larger numbers of students being assessed at any one time, finding a standard is simpler. (And so, reliability of marking can be achieved more quickly than in a clinical setting.) But as with any assessment, accuracy is improved by seeing a range of performances by the same student.

• The demonstration of overall professional performance is much broader than in an academic assessment which targets specific skills to evaluate at any one time. Personal value judgements can influence the weighting given to each part of the clinical perform- ance and may affect the overall judgement of the performance. Therapists must therefore be aware of their own biases and check with the weighting agreed by the school and adjust their judgement accordingly.

• The fear of failing a student is more personally demanding in the clinical environment than in an academic setting where students are often marked anonymously.

Trying to make the criteria more specific and performance-related, as I did when advising in my role as clinical instructor, will not necessarily address these issues. No wonder we were all uncomfort- able with this. For example, a more intimate relationship with the student modifies judgement both positively and negatively, and may in fact be more accurate (closer to the truth about the student's real ability) than any judgement made when the student is one of many in the academic setting. It is important then to recognise that biases may arise as a result of these problems – or even from others yet unspecified, for example some that might be personal to the therapist.

Student assessment in undergraduate programmes

Following my masters degree, I joined the Bachelor of Science in physiotherapy degree programme at McMaster University as a lecturer and moved from the field of clinical education and assess- ment into the academic world. I co-ordinated the rehabilitation course. For the assessment, students wrote an essay about a rehabilitation issue of choice (that is, no two students wrote on the same topic). In marking my first set of essays, I gave a 'B+' to one student – 78 per cent, which was based on some loosely defined criteria, handed down to me by the previous course co-ordinator. The student appealed against my mark and asked for a re-read. (She wanted to get into a masters programme and needed straight 'A's in her work – that is, 80 per cent or above). She requested definitive evidence of the two marks that put her paper at a 'B' grade instead of an 'A' grade. I re-read the paper but did not change my mark. (So, was this proof that I was consistent with my own judgement?!) Because the student again appealed against my mark, the previous course co-ordinator was asked to read the paper. She said that, in her opinion, it was worth an 'A'. Her comments on the quality of the student's writing echoed mine and we agreed on where the student could have improved. But she maintained it was an 'A' paper, and I a 'B'. Whose opinion was correct? She had had more experience than I in marking written papers and she claimed that it was an 'A' paper. Although I was now quite experienced in marking the professional performance of students in the clinical environment, I had had little experience at evaluating students academic achievements. I was now in a university programme and was having to 'feel my way' through a different set of assessment rules that judged the rigour of scholarly thought. In the end, we awarded the student the required 'A'.

I was left angry and confused by the incident. I was hurt and upset that my professional judgement had been overridden by another's that could not be clearly articulated. Questioning the validity of our judgement I was unnerved that perhaps we were influenced by the assertiveness of the student's protest. How often do evaluators sway a few marks (up or down), when a student is known to them and especially when there are foreboding consequences to the mark (for instance failing a student, knowing that they will have to stay down a year, repeat a clinical placement etc.).

Insight (4)

I had come from a professional environment into an academic institution, where the expectations of students had changed. I was in a situation where I had to evaluate scholarly activity with only a clinically based professional frame of reference on which to base my judgements. I was unfamiliar with how to mark written assessments and further, I was wrestling with how they related to clinical practice. Evidence indicated that written assessments did not predict professional competence (Dunn et al., 1985).

What I had failed to grasp in my defensiveness was my need to develop the academic skills needed to assess undergraduate degree work. In moving towards professional autonomy, physiotherapy had recognised the need for an expanded theoretical base. Intellectually, I embraced the changes, but, the only model of physiotherapy assessment that I knew was based on my experiences in clinical areas. I was therefore trying to mark papers with a clinical hat on.

As in any professional practice, there is a large element of tacit knowledge in the practice of education. A knowledge that comes with experience, that cannot necessarily be articulated (Brew, 1993). My understanding of the academic environment had not been developed and that was quite evident when it came to the assessment of those scholastic qualities and thinking processes. Yelloly (1995) indicates that tacit knowledge is acquired 'only through repeated familiarity with the actual experience'. Thus, with repeated experience (particularly when accompanied by reflection) an educator can develop skill and confidence in assessing student performance and the criteria become internalised. Due to her prior experience at marking papers, the second evaluator of the student's paper had developed insights that were not apparent to a novice such as myself at that time. Perhaps if I had known this, my course of action would have been different. I might have tried to give myself as much experience at marking (old) papers and discussed discrepancies in marks with the more experienced examiner. Instead I made sure that for the following year there were some very clear guidelines for assessing the students' written work in the hope of avoiding this kind of incident again. This was particularly important since I had enrolled more examiners to ease the burden of marking. I needed to know that each examiner was marking consistently. The inter-rater reliability exercises were helped considerably by the development of the specific marking criteria.

Insight (5)

Still wrestling in my mind about the value of defining standards of performance, I was excited to find an article by Usherwood *et al.* (1995) in which they described how criteria generated for the assessment of clinical practice in medicine were no longer being used effectively. By involving tutors and students in the revision of the standard competencies, consistency between markers improved. Perhaps these more explicit competencies for marking were more comprehensive and sophisticated than the previous ones and therefore more relevant and easier to assess. Perhaps, on the other hand, the improvement was due to the opportunity that the team of assessors had to explore their values and make explicit some of their biases. I wonder what is the value of developed criteria, particularly specific, behaviourally related criteria, if the people carrying out the assessment have not been party to the process of developing the criteria? In my example, it might have been the clarity of the criteria established that enhanced the inter-rater reliability. However, the consistency of marking was due, more likely, to the opportunity to discuss and use the criteria under controlled conditions first.

Continuing the story

With these experiences behind me which had encouraged me to tighten the structure around my assessments, and with the need for greater accountability in higher education, I spent the next six years at McMaster developing performance-based criteria against which students could be marked. I prided myself on developing excellent inter-rater reliability agreement based on well-defined criteria, model answers and evaluator training exercises (Chapman *et al.*, 1993). I joined two national committees to develop standards for Canadian Physiotherapy Qualifying Exams. We were asked to design examinations that would ensure a minimum standard of practice from the graduates of all Canadian schools and would discriminate between many overseas applicants applying for work status in Canada. We chose and developed the very structured Multiple Choice Question examination for its ability to evaluate knowledge, and Objective Structured Clinical Examinations to measure practical abilities and professional attitudes. The inter-rater reliability scores were getting better because each exam had specific criteria that could be measured! I could more confidently justify the mark I allocated a student for a piece of work. Despite all this, I still questioned whether I was evaluating the professional attitudes and critical thinking abilities well enough to discriminate between students with professional qualities and those who were merely technically competent?

Insight (6)

My discomfort with assessment at one level was being resolved. I was being swept (enthusiastically, because defining competencies and standards fitted my need for an assessment security blanket) by the political tide of being accountable.

We had a responsibility to the public to establish a standard of practice that was outcome-based (achieved by graduates before they could be licensed to practise).

Strongly adhering to the principles of positivism (Hartley, 1992), I traded the assessment of professional competence involving professional judgements adapted to unique situations (Jones and Joss, 1995) for reproducibility and discrimination on technical merit.

Assessment at the University of Southampton

In 1992 I joined the School of Occupational Therapy and Physiotherapy at the University of Southampton when the under-graduate programme was being designed and validated. I became co-ordinator of assessments for the programmes and was respons-ible for helping to choose assessment methods and develop standards of marking. There was a constant tension for me, in trying to develop assessments that:

- evaluated students' creativity, critical thinking, clinical reasoning, ability to argue (all skills worthy of the kind of graduate expected from an honours degree programme);

- discriminated between students and gave those students who were capable, a chance to excel;
- were reliable and could be used by a variety of staff to make similar judgements about the level of work of the student.

Since many of the school staff were new to education and because of my own past experiences, I erred on the side of establishing an assessment system that would be unambiguous and reliable. Most assessment instruments had carefully designed criteria for assessment and inter-rater reliability exercises were set up to improve the accuracy of the marking.

These tightly controlled assessments resulted in a very small spread of marks, with only a few students showing excellence by achieving the top grades. The more explicit the criteria for assessment the smaller the range of marks. Interestingly, physiotherapists seemed to be more comfortable with the concept of competency-based assessment. The clinical reasoning used by physiotherapists followed an identifiable pattern and there are many definable clinical performance skills to be evaluated. The occupational therapists had more difficulty defining performance-related competencies. Assessing their professional skills required the assessment of more abstract qualities.

Insight (7)

On reflection, I wonder whether the reason that these competency-based assessments lacked the power to discriminate between students was because we had defined only one level of competency. We had not known how to categorise the students. If they achieved the criteria, did that then warrant an 'A' grade, or was what we had developed an indication of an average performance ('C' grade)? If the latter was the case, what then did the student have to do to achieve an 'A'? (Please don't tell me that I have another set of criteria to develop – I'm exhausted with trying to define at one level only!)

Perhaps, our competencies had failed to capture those more abstract elements of critical thinking, application and professional qualities that would have allowed us to discriminate between students.

I then looked at the differences in their response to the assessment process from the two professional groups in the school.

Physiotherapy evolved from a Medical Model of care (Hagedorn, 1992; Thomas-Edding, 1993; Turnbull, 1994). The thinking behind the approach is quite linear (hypothetico-deductive) (Higgs, 1992a). A trigger (case presentation) generates a series of hypotheses in the mind of the practitioner. (The quantity and sophistication of the hypothesis usually determines the accuracy of the eventual diagnosis: Elstein, 1978.) The assessment process follows a fairly predictable path designed to confirm (or refute) the initial hypothesis. 'What you are looking for determines what you see' (Polan, 1988, p. 103). Once a diagnosis is established, then a treatment can be initiated based on that diagnosis (often regardless of individual patient characteristics or social situation). The practitioner is trying to see the unique circumstances before him or her as an example of a general case (see Golby, 1993). This method of reasoning is reductionist. It is evident not only in diagnosing a patient's problem but it is transferred to other professional activities. It stands to reason then that the type of assessment of professional performance that best suits medicine and related disciplines is one that is logical in approach and based on observable features that fit into recognisable patterns of behaviour. (This emulates the clinical reasoning practised in the clinical environment.) A competency-based assessment scheme seems to fit favourably with the learned pattern of making judgements.

Occupational therapy originated from outside the medical profession (Fleming, 1991). In the assessment and management of clients, hypothetical reasoning is only one of several reasoning processes employed. They frequently use continuous reasoning, involving revisions of decisions when further evidence has accumulated, and reflections on clients' responses to the therapeutic process (Law *et al.*, 1995). This allows therapists to resolve issues that were initially unclear, or live with the uncertainty of being unable to predict an outcome, because of the influence of individual variables. Perhaps this is why the occupational therapists in our school feel more constrained by the specific criteria in performance-based competencies and less threatened or insecure when the issues are equivocal or abstract.

Critical incident

My critical incident centred on the assessment in a module that I co-ordinated, called 'Teaching and Learning', for the Year One occupational therapy and physiotherapy students. In small groups, students gave a ten minute presentation to other students and examiners, the students summarised their approach, justifying it and discussing the limitations. Since the module focused on students developing self-directed learning skills I felt it imperative that the students be involved in negotiating the assessment criteria for the presentation of their work. In a workshop, students established a list of items that would be evaluated. I then organised the list into discrete sections, placing weightings against each section, so that students were then clear about what was being evaluated and how each section contributed to their overall mark. In my mind, these criteria would illustrate the students' competency in their presentation skills and their understanding of the principles and application of module content. Since the students had these very clearly defined criteria ahead of time, there would be no 'playing examination games'. Assessing them would be a piece of cake. This would alleviate my anxiety and that of my fellow examiners. By using the criteria we would minimise the discrepancy in our marking and would be able to justify clearly the mark we gave to the student. (In fact, the students would be able to evaluate their own performance and would therefore be able to anticipate, fairly accurately, what their mark would be, which would not only diminish their disappointment at a low mark but also reduce the examiners' worry of having to respond to angry students who had expected better marks.) Eventually, after years at the game, I felt I had arrived at the solution that would end all tension! Why was it then, that when we came to mark the presentations

- there were still discrepancies between the markers on the performance of the same group of students;
- there were still pairs of examiners that marked their students more harshly (or more leniently) than others;
- there were more 'A's than in the assessments for other modules;
- the majority of students (66 per cent!) inaccurately marked themselves as having achieved an 'A' standard for their performance?

The students were most upset too. Even though they had helped to establish the marking criteria, they had not all achieved the 'A' they had expected as a result of explicitly knowing what they were required to do ahead of time!

My personal disappointment lay in not being able to give those students who were innovative in their presentation, a different mark from others, because the criteria did not cater for that uniqueness.

I was mystified, disappointed and quite angry at the failure of the assessment to resolve my dilemma. I really felt I had 'captured it' and despite all my efforts to make the criteria explicit, the exercise left me feeling like a novice educator. I was 'hauled up' (in the nicest possible way!) by the external examiners who recommended that *I* take responsibility for establishing the marking criteria; that our criteria would constitute a 'C' grade only and that we should use graded guidelines developed in the department of Occupational Therapy at University College of Ripon and York, St John's to grade the superior performances of the students. Although I recognised why they had advocated doing it, I was not happy with this at all. It took away some of the control that the students could exercise over their learning process and we would be back to interpreting the assessment guidelines, thus potentially reducing again inter-rater reliability and the assessment's accuracy.

I ran the assessment again four months later on the second group of first year students. The range of marks was still skewed (was this because marks are always higher for a presentation assessment than a written one?) and clustered (showing little discrimination between the performance of the groups). Inter-rater reliability was no better than before, and students were still disappointed in their marks, though their self-assessments were slightly more accurate!

I was left feeling betrayed. All this effort to establish a better system of assessment and it had not worked! Surely, one needed clear criteria for assessment to improve consistency, yet as soon as this was done, assessment of the unique qualities of individual students was lost. Even if abstract features were highlighted in the criteria, interpretation of them was difficult and led to increased pressures on the examiners to agree and be congruent with their marking.

I started to lose confidence in my ability as an educator and as co-ordinator of assessments in the Occupational Therapy/Physiotherapy programme. After all, I was encouraging other staff to establish criteria for assessment, in an attempt to ensure reliability and accuracy of marking. Where was I going wrong? There was something wrong with my thinking – yet the literature and my experiences all supported my attempts to specify criteria for assessment. I was being challenged to open up and use an assessment system that incorporated acknowledgement of the abstract, intangible elements of performance. My attempts to define these into measurable elements was failing desperately. What should I do?

I talked at length to one of the external examiners who shed some light on my dilemma and started to restore my confidence. She was an American and in discussing the two cultures (North American and British) explained how there was a fundamental difference in thinking between the two countries. In America there is support for a philosophy of 'Positivism' which is more mechanistic or reductionist in its point of view. This Post-Modernist (Pietroni, 1995) perspective has been slower to evolve in the United Kingdom. The 'interpretative or heuristic' underpinning has allowed UK examiners to embrace the subjectivity of assessment more easily. An article in the *Times Higher Educational Supplement* (Eiland, 1995) further supported the line of thinking on this. It described how the standard of marking in the United States was becoming alarmingly inflated. There emerged an insistence that all things are (to be seen to be) equal. But in an attempt to remove the negative effects of competition and foster collaboration, an essential part of the assessment system seemed to have been removed. This is shown in the Harvard University figure, where 83.6 per cent of the senior students graduated with honours. The author claimed that in addition to the political correctness, economics were forcing the marking up spuriously. Good grades mean better occupational opportunities. Therefore, families who are paying large university fees expect and do not tolerate anything but a top mark.

Insight (8)

I have only managed to explore the influence of the difference in my cultural underpinnings a little. It would take a degree in sociology to fully understand all the implications! The attitude towards assessment, however, does appear to be significantly different in these two cultures. Canada's drive for professional accountability has followed the steps of the United States in developing competencies or defined standards of practice for graduates to achieve. This means that, within that system, allegedly all graduates could succeed and given time and the correct learning strategies, all could acquire 'A's. This is in contrast to the British system, where the honours degree classification warrants norm-referenced student marking. That is, that students are marked compared with one another.

Another difference I noticed when I first joined the University in Southampton was that I would mark students from a 'full pot', deducting marks when I perceived an error or omission. My English colleagues would be 'filling the pot up' as they went; only giving a student a mark when they perceived that the student had earned it. This difference in perception led to a great discrepancy in the marking of the same paper, with my way generating a mark that was consistently a grade higher than my colleagues. I could, however, through my experience, more or less justify every mark I had subtracted if I had been made accountable! Clearly this was the product of being involved in a criterion-based system of marking where one could more easily detect what was omitted from the performance than count up all the pieces of the performance that could justify a mark. I felt remarkably freer when thinking that perhaps the differences in culture contributed to my assessment approach – and that it was not simply my poor standard as an educator. I still have not fully resolved the tensions between the two approaches to assessment but I am learning to live with unanswered questions and am exploring different ways of conducting assessments in a more open manner.

Reflections and conclusions

The process of concluding

I have been struggling for a few weeks now to conclude my story. I have been thinking: "all this reading, all this thinking, all this energy, and what do I have to show for it?" Just a few related incidents? So what do I make of them now and how will my attitude towards student assessments change in the future as a result of writing this chapter? Well, the answer is not entirely clear and I expect the revelations will continue to occur as I continue to reflect on assessments in the future. But right now, I have put the following ideas together.

There are no clear answers to assessing physiotherapy students. The profession is evolving rapidly and what is suitable today will not necessarily be suitable tomorrow (Turnbull, 1994). What is suitable in one field is not necessarily suitable in another (for example, institution versus community, academic versus clinical environment). We therefore have to live with uncertainty, and work to develop assessment schemes that are flexible to evolve with the changes.

When I return to my initial question of fairness at the expense of accuracy, there is a justifiable tension based, it seems, on professional orientation, educational experience and personal biases. The answer lies somewhere in between the confining, reductionist, structure of competencies and the enigmatic and ambiguous world of conjectural assessment. However, to find this ideal situation it is vital to take into account the expertise of the educator and make allowances for individual interpretation of guidelines put in place to elucidate the process expected of the students. When I looked back over the incidents I felt there was a progression in my ability to assess the students; however, at the time, my progress was masked and confounded by my not recognising the evolution of the profession and the more drastic effect of the change in physiotherapy education when it moved from its clinically based teaching in hospital units to the university. Based on this new understanding, a couple of weeks ago, I thought that there must be a difference in the way that educators approach the task of student assessment, that depends on their level of experience, not on whether or not clear standards of expected practice have been defined. (After all, I was a seasoned assessor and still had difficulty coming to any agreement with my fellow markers in my critical incident even though we had clearly defined criteria for assessment of performance.)

Investigating this line of thought, I can now parallel my progress over the years with the stages of Dreyfus and Dreyfus's (1986) Model of Skill Acquisition. This model has been applied to the development of clinical reasoning skills in occupational therapy

(Slater and Cohn, 1991). What the model suggests is that as a novice, performance is constrained by limited experience. Thus the inexperienced educator needs more structure and specific guidelines in order to judge student performance. By participating in the development of guiding criteria, the novice may develop his or her academic judgement and have something concrete on which to base his or her judgement. (My experience in clinical supervision and in the initial university setting.) As experience is gained, so the more proficient educator will judge the performance or essay or presentation 'as a whole rather than as isolated parts' (Slater and Cohn, 1991). The need for the student's performance to be subdivided into measurable components is reduced, until, as an expert with much experience, intuitive judgements about performance can be made with minimal reference to more abstract guidelines.

Here I want to add a word of caution. A thought occurred to me when I was reflecting on my need as a novice to have clearer guidelines for assessment. Although my intentions were honourable in setting up clear criteria for assessments, I could have been encouraging the students to develop superficial learning habits. This would have been quite contrary to the outcome that I had desired. In focusing on achieving the competencies the students may have inadvertently employed superficial learning strategies to accomplish the tasks. They would simply demonstrate a performance without necessarily reflecting on the purpose or the process. In breaking down performance into discrete elements for observation the student would learn bits and not pay attention to the integration or application of the component parts. If competencies are used in assessment therefore, due consideration must be given to the process of learning employed by the student.

The understanding that I have developed as a result of the insights, subsequent investigation and overall reflection on my experiences will influence how I set up my assessments in the future. When I select my guidelines for assessment, the depth and concreteness of them will depend on the needs (based on experiences and personal characteristics) of my team of assessors, as well as my own level of experience with the assessment format and level of student education. It is critical to develop consistency between markers – inter-rater reliability (or myself on different occasions – intra-rater reliability). To achieve this in the past, I have developed more structured guidelines, to restrict evaluators exercising their personal biases when evaluating. Whereas some guidelines lend clarity, over-prescribing the criteria precludes assessing critical parts of the academic or practical performance. Whereas before I was appre-hensive about looking at and sharing my own biases, lest I be found wanting, I now think it crucial to introduce this exploration formally into the assessment process. The more each person understands his or her bias and accepts the subjectivity that will influence his or her assessment the fairer and more consistent those judgements will be (Tversky and Kahneman, 1974). Inter-rater reliability exercises are an integral part of our school system, but the emphasis is on getting to the right mark rather than to understanding the process of discovering personal influences on decisions.

In addition to exploring the question of the reliability and valid-ity of student assessments, I wanted to draw a parallel in my conclusions to clinical practice in physiotherapy. I think that the issues of assessment are similar whether it is a student or a client that is being assessed. In the current climate of service contracts and conspicuous accountability measures, there has been a shift towards using standardised assessment forms, the results of which can be easily fed into a computer data base in order to compare services, approaches and outcomes. This appears to improve the reliability of clinical assessments and client progress. General-isability is also enhanced so client groups can be compared for favourable outcomes. But the individual problems and unique features of each client are lost in the quest for quality assurance. Physiotherapists are faced with a similar dilemma to that found in the academic environment, where the desire for fair judgement conflicts with the assessment of individual characteristics, which influence performance.

Insight (9)

There are no straightforward answers, though for many years I thought that the competency-based assessment was the structure that was needed to dispel the uncertainty. Added to which, because I was so aware of how poor marks could affect a person, as an evaluator I wanted all students to succeed. (The competency-based system with its focus on explicit criteria seemed to give students the best chance. And, when starting with a full pot and emptying it, it seemed more likely that the pot would not get below the half-way mark.) Perhaps this also goes a little way to explaining why there is a greater chance of success in North America, which condones the criterion-based system of marking. With these insights, improved self-esteem and recognition that no one has the answer, that we are all struggling with these fundamental assessment issues and that what suits one person or one system may not necessarily suit another, I can pursue my academic and clinical career with more confidence and a better tolerance of uncertainty.

My hope is that if you are willing to try this process, you too will come to a level of understanding with your ability to assess others, recognising the tensions and being aware of the imperfections of the system, and be able to work out a 'modus operandi' that suits your situation.

References

Bloom, B. S. (ed.) (1974). *Taxonomy of Educational Objectives: the Classification of Educational Goals.* David McKay.

Boud, D., Cohen, R. and Walker, D. (1993). Introduction: Understanding learning from experience. In *Using Experience for Learning* (D. Boud, R. Cohen and D. Walker, eds.), pp. 36–56. The Society for Research into Higher Education & Open University Press.

Brew, A. (1993). Unlearning through experience. In *Using Experience for Learning* (D. Boud, R. Cohen and D. Walker, eds.), pp. 95–108. The Society for Research into Higher Education & Open University Press.

Chapman, J. A., Westmorland, M. G., Norman, G. R. *et al.* (1993). The structured oral self-directed learning evaluation: one method of evaluating the clinical reasoning skills of occupational therapy and physiotherapy students. *Medical Teacher*, 15, 223–236.

Dreyfus, H. L. and Dreyfus, S. E. (1986). *Mind Over Machine.* Free Press.

Dunn, W. R., Hamilton, D. D. and Harden, R. M. (1985). Techniques of identifying competencies needed of doctors. *Medical Teacher*, 7, 15–25.

Eiland, M. A. (1995). American gripes about grades. *Times Higher Education Supplement*, 11 August, p. 13.

Elstein, A. L. (1978). *Medical Problem Solving: an Analysis of Clinical Reasoning.* Harvard University Press.

Fish, D. (1989). *Learning Through Practice in Initial Teacher Training: a Challenge for the Partners.* Kogan Page.

Fish, D. (1991). But can you prove it? Quality assurance and the reflective practitioner. *Assessment and Evaluation in Higher Education*, 16, 22–36.

Fish, D. (1996). Values, competency-based training and teacher education. In *Values in Teacher Education*, Volume 2 (C. Selmes and W. Robb, eds.), pp. 44–50. National Association of Values in Education.

Fleming, M. H. (1991). Clinical reasoning in medicine compared with clinical reasoning in occupational therapy. *American Journal of Occupational Therapy*, **45**, 988–1005.

Golby, M. (1993). *Case Study as Educational Research*. Fair Way Publications.

Hagedorn, R. (1992). *Occupational Therapy: Foundations for Practice Models, Frames of Reference and Core Skills*. Churchill Livingstone.

Hartley, D. (1992). Teacher appraisal: a policy analysis. In *Professional Issues in Education* (G. Kirk and R. Glaister, eds.), pp. 52–53. Scottish Academic Press.

Higgs, J. (1992a). Developing clinical reasoning competencies. *Physiotherapy*, **78**, 575–581.

Higgs, J. (1992b). Managing clinical education: the educator-manager and the self-directed learner. *Physiotherapy*, **78**, 822–828.

Jones, S. and Joss, R. (1995). Models of professionalism. In *Learning and Teaching in Social Work: Towards Reflective Practice* (M. Yelloly and M. Henkel, eds.), pp. 15–33. Jessica Kingsley Publishers.

Knowles, M. (1975). *Self-Directed Learning: a Guide for Learners and Teachers*. Follett Pub. Co.

Law, M., Baptiste, S. and Mills, J. (1995). Client-centred practice: What does it mean and does it make a difference? *Canadian Journal of Occupational Therapy*, **62**, 250–257.

Mager, R. (1975). *Preparing Instructional Objectives* (2nd Edn), Fearon-Pitman Publishers.

Norman, G. R., Van der Vleuten, C. P. M. and De Graaff, E. (1991). Pitfalls in the pursuit of objectivity: issues of validity, efficiency and acceptability. *Medical Education*, **25**, 119–126.

Pietroni, M. (1995). The nature and aims of professional education for social workers: a postmodern perspective. In *Learning and Teaching in Social Work: Towards Reflective Practice* (M. Yelloly and M. Henkel, eds.), pp. 44–46. Jessica Kingsley Publishers.

Polan, A. (1988). Assessing the future. In *Turning Teaching into Learning* (D. Fish, ed.), West London Press.

Postel, D. (1993). Putting the heart back into learning. In *Using Experience for Learning* (D. Boud, R. Cohen and D. Walker, eds.), pp. 123–144. The Society for Research into Higher Education & Open University Press.

Race, P. (1995). The art of assessing 1, *The New Academic: the Magazine of Teaching and Learning in Higher Education*, **4**, 3–6.

Schön, D. A. (1987). *Educating the Reflective Practitioner*. Jossey-Bass.

Shepard, K. F. and Jensen, G. M. (1990). Physical therapist curricula for the 1990s: educating the reflective practitioner. *Physical Therapy*, **70**, 566–577.

Slater, D. Y. and Cohn, E. S. (1991). Staff development through analysis of practice. *American Journal of Occupational Therapy*, **45**, 1038–1044.

Thomas-Edding, D. (1993). Physiotherapy curriculum: transition from diploma to degree. *Physiotherapy Canada*, **45**, 9–12.

Turnbull, G. I. (1994). Educating tomorrow's colleagues: the physiotherapist in the university system. *Physiotherapy Canada*, **46**, 9–14.

Tversky, A. and Kahneman, D. (1974). Judgement under uncertainty: heuristics and biases. *Science*, **185**, 1124–1131.

Usherwood, T., Challis, M., Joesbury, H. and Hannay, D. (1995). Competence-based summative assessment of a student-directed course: involvement of key stakeholders. *Medical Education*, **29**, 144–149.

Yelloly, M. (1995). Professional competence and higher education. In *Learning and Teaching in Social Work: Towards Reflective Practice* (M. Yelloly and M. Henkel, eds.), pp. 123–144. Jessica Kingsley Publishers.

Chapter 10

Responding to being touched

Clive Andrewes

Introduction

This chapter sets out to investigate the process by which professional judgement was explored by a group of nurses in clinical practice. The practitioners, through a variety of approaches, including a reflective practice group, examined how they knew, or chose, appropriate responses when they were touched or held, while caring for people with dementia. The chapter is not designed to give an in-depth understanding of touch, or of reflective practice. Instead it narrates the story of how, in the hectic and messy world of clinical practice, insights and understanding into professional judgement were developed. It is written from the perspective of the lecturer who facilitates the work of the group, and it primarily explores my thoughts and feelings on this journey of returning to clinical practice.

The chapter describes the background to the journey, the path that was followed and comments on insights and ideas that were developed during this exploration. In the first section of the chapter, short passages which are subtitled 'comment' are included. These contain thoughts and reflections on the particular part of the story that is being told. The second section of the story is described using Van Manen's (1990) phenomenological approach to thinking. This allows for a narrative to be told, while at the same time reflecting on the byways and paths that a story generates.

Background

Nursing, as a practice-focused discipline, is undergoing major transformation in its understanding of the theoretical foundation and conceptual underpinning of its practice. The reasons for this are complex. They are intricately involved with nursing's continuing exploration of the basis of nursing as a discipline in its own right, the articulation of nursing's unique role within an inter-professional health care team, the struggle to understand what is clinically effective in our practice and debate about how we exercise our professional judgement in the care that we give.

These general themes were given a powerful impetus by Benner's work (1984), *From Novice to Expert*. This work explored the knowledge embedded in clinical nursing practice. This was done within the framework of examining the transition of a qualified practitioner from novice to an expert. She argued that the features of clinical expertise exhibited by experts are 'an in-depth knowledge of a clinical population; advanced recognitional abilities; and increased use of past whole situations or situation specific referents for understanding the clinical situation' (1984. p. 42). This work, and her view of expert practice, has been highly influential within nursing. It appeared to a number of nurses that if we could achieve more clarity on the basis of expert practice, then we would achieve further understanding of the broader questions we were asking about professional judgement.

In exploring expert practice, nursing has been heavily influenced by Schön's (1983) seminal work on reflective practice. This was published a year before Benner's work, and there appears, within nursing, to have been a synthesis of these two approaches. As a result, reflective practice is attracting considerable debate within nursing education and practice.

Over the past ten years nursing literature has highlighted the need to promote the concept of reflective practice and to assist students in reflection. This is demonstrated by authors such as Clarke (1986), Powell (1989), Johns (1995), Lumby (1991), Reed and Proctor (1993) and Street (1991). The purpose of this approach is to 'enable the practitioner to access, understand and learn through his or her lived experiences and, as a consequence, to take congruent action towards developing increasing effectiveness within the context of what is understood as desirable practice' (Johns, 1995, p. 231).

As a result of this movement, nursing curricula abound with reflective practice groups, reflective practice assignments, analyses of critical incidents, reflective journals and diaries. In practice settings, qualified practitioners may be involved in action learning groups examining issues of professional practice. In addition, all practitioners are required to keep a portfolio related to their continuing professional development which can be used as a basis for continuing registration. These portfolios may include a section where the practitioner has reflected upon and critically analysed their own practice.

This move into reflective practice is not without its critics. Kottkamp reminds us that 'Reflection and reflective practice may become only the latest in the casualty list of ideas with great potential that have been reduced to the level of tinkling jargon through uninformed use' (Kottkamp, 1990, p. 200). Greenwood argues that 'too often reflective practice uses espoused theories rather than theories in use (theories which actually govern practice)' (Greenwood, 1993, p. 1185). Also, and perhaps critically, she wonders if some of the methods advocated by Schön failed to confront the 'messy, indeterminate situations of uncertainty; instability; uniqueness and value conflict' in the practice of nursing.

This background of interest in this approach to learning, its usefulness in exploring expert practice and how practitioners exercise judgement, has led to lecturers in nursing becoming involved in this process.

Comment

On a personal note, it is interesting to realise the importance of this background. The culture within nursing and education was changing, which created the opportunity for this particular exploration. How much harder, or more lonely, it is for people to develop and explore their own theories, when the culture or organisation is at variance with our personal theories. However, the tension that the latter situation causes can perhaps be creative. Many ideas have been developed across a range of academic disciplines, against a background of resistance. The emphasis in the present health and social care climate of measurable outcomes is a backcloth which is causing tension but has also stimulated the creative exploration of professional judgement.

Personal involvement in reflective practice through education

As a nurse, now primarily involved in education, I have been involved in reflective practice groups in a number of ways. This has occurred through working with pre- and post-registration nurses on degree schemes who use reflective practice groups to facilitate the integration of practice and theory. These provide a method to discover, analyse and critique the complex processes involved in professional practice.

This approach was also used to facilitate discussion between groups of qualified nurses within practice settings. Qualified practitioners explored the conceptual base of their practice, identifying the concepts that underpin that practice, the values and skills that they used in their practice and how they exercised their professional judgement. This approach was seen as a 'partnership between academic nurses and nurse clinicians to begin to tackle the issues that are currently affecting nursing's ability to demonstrate its effectiveness in meeting today's health care need' (Graham, 1996, p. 265).

The journey

One such group of practitioners were mental health nurses working within a development unit for nursing the elderly mentally ill. This group met every Friday afternoon on their ward to explore their practice in order to gain deeper understanding of the knowledge and skills they used to care for older people who were acutely mentally ill. My role was to facilitate discussion in the group. It was involvement with this particular group that was the trigger to this particular journey.

Comment

This involvement, which I wanted, was again made easier by a number of factors. Firstly, it was made easy by the refusal and reluctance of many lecturers to explore this approach to education. Consequently, my desire to facilitate the work of reflective groups was not only welcomed but enabled some other lecturers to breathe a sigh of relief that they were not now going to be asked to help. One typical comment was "I was terrified they might ask me!" Secondly, the creation of nursing development units supported a culture where the practitioners were enthusiastic about exploring their practice. So not only was the general milieu changing but my local university and nursing was also subject to this change.

Windows of opportunity existed. These windows allowed the possibility of the journey. There were some travellers who wished to explore the subterranean terrain of their practice. How marvellous this was. In many instances, the persuasion, nudging and cajoling needed can be exhausting. So much so, that one may easily give up.

Reflective practice groups

The group in question was one of a number that as a group of academics we had been working with to clarify the issues referred to earlier. Initially this work had been based on exploring their practice through Graham's conceptual framework. This framework consists of reflecting upon: the purpose of nursing work/practice; nursing roles; nursing activities; concepts of caring; fundamental work; aim of the work; resources to do the work; and the care delivery system (Graham, 1996).

The particular focus of this work that led to my personal stimulation to explore an aspect of my own practice was the reflection on the concepts underpinning caring.

The mental health group

The practitioners in the mental health group had identified a number of concepts that they wished to explore in their own practice. These included: hope, helplessness, support, dignity, embarrassment, humour and touch. It was the exploration of the concept and use of touch in their practice that was the focus for this particular voyage into my own practice.

Comment

The micro concepts underpinning caring had been, and remain, an area of considerable personal and academic interest. I had started exploring these within formal educational delivery through leading a module on 'Carenology'. This was aimed at exploring caring in professional practice. The title of the module, which caused a variety of reactions, mostly unfavourable, was chosen to highlight the increasing scholarship in this approach to understanding nursing. A module entitled 'The art and science of caring' was never commented upon. Words are so important and convey so many different messages.

To some degree I undoubtedly influenced the practitioners to use micro concepts as a way of illuminating their understanding. This was not necessarily wrong but there was a potential danger that my very formative personal theory in relation to these concepts was uncritically accepted. In developing views and a theoretical perspective, the challenge to that perspective is crucial in helping its clarification. In developing my own theory of judgement and its relationship to caring I was at an instinctive stage of what I thought seemed a way forward to explaining expert practice. We need others to help and challenge us in this exploration, otherwise we reinforce our own views. Thinking and theory can then become a means of defending an entrenched position, rather than creatively exploring new pathways to explain the subterranean world of professional practice.

The group's reflection on touch

Over the previous weeks we had discussed the concepts of hope, hopelessness and humour. It was now the turn of touch!

The discussion within the group in relation to touch revealed a number of themes. The word 'revealed' is deliberately used, as the conclusions arrived at were not evident at first but came to light, or to the surface, through analytical reflection. The *first* related to the forms of touch that the practitioners used within a nurse–patient relationship. The agreed view was that touch could not be understood by identifying its components or dimensions. The feeling was that touch should be seen as all pervasive within a relationship. This bears out Weiss's (1979) idea of touch as a complex *gestalt*.

The *second* theme that emerged was in relation to a discussion of the use of touch with people who were restless and confused within this practice setting. The behaviour that can be present is when people 'clutch' or 'grab you', either as they are walking by a nurse or as a nurse is walking by them – a common feature within this area of practice.

The expert practitioners were surprised to realise that they felt they knew that the person needed different things from the nurse according to the form of touching behaviour. They were surprised in the sense that they had not realised this overtly, although their practice demonstrated expertise or artistry or intuitive knowing. So how did they respond differently?

One form of touch meant the person wanted a physical need met such as food, water, or assistance with elimination. A second form of touch meant there was a need for comfort in relation to distress and a person required hugging or holding warmly. A third form of touch arose from people feeling lost and uncertain. The person could require 'being with the nurse', or 'holding on to the nurse'. This entailed walking with the nurse around the unit while remaining in physical contact with the nurse. This they termed 'anchoring touch'.

Some of the members of the groups knew which form of intervention was needed, while others knew of the range of interventions available but needed a trial and error approach to identify what was effective. So on what basis did the practitioners exercise their judgement?

The participants decided that they wished to explore this concept in more detail before moving on to other areas. The reasons for this seem to relate to their feeling that they had developed, in the words of one practitioner, "real insight into an area of practice I had not thought about". This motivated them to continue to explore this area of practice.

Comment

The term 'anchoring touch' does not seem novel. Yet it is not in the literature. It did make instant sense to the practitioners. One wonders to what extent the fact that the language of formal theory is not derived from practitioners, means that the theory itself may be disregarded. So do we need to develop a richer, or newer language to describe the artistry of expert practice?

My own reasons for exploration into 'being touched'

Touch may be a small and not significant aspect of care to some people. However, I would argue it is of critical importance. It provided a vehicle to develop my understanding of how we exercise our judgement in a professional caring relationship. This understanding would naturally be relevant to other areas where skilled judgement is required.

In caring for people who are distressed, restless and agitated and who can be in a twilight world of their own, what is the aim of the care we are providing? A critical aspect must surely include the relief of distress, the promotion of comfort, meeting physical need, imparting a sense of belonging and feelings of safety. The skilled judgement of the use of the appropriate form of touch will undoubtedly play a key role in helping to achieve these goals.

A further reason why touch was of particular interest to me relates to uncovering the 'invisibility' of nursing. I have been influenced by Lawler's (1991) powerful work, *Behind the Screens: Nursing, Somology and the Problem of the Body*. This examined a whole area of practice which had been highly private. The richness of her findings illustrates the importance of uncovering the hidden world of much of our practice.

The problem of our 'hidden world' is compounded by the difficulty of understanding expert practice in areas where a limited range of technologies and procedures are used. As Sutton and Smith argue:

> In these settings, each nursing situation occurs in the private realm of the nurse–client interaction and predominantly requires a focus on the personhood of the client. The work, therefore, of each practitioner is invisible and unknown to others. This invisibility makes it difficult if not impossible to recognise and acknowledge expertness in these less technological settings. (Sutton and Smith, 1995, p. 1039)

Comment

It is in these invisible areas that expertise is demonstrated. The skills to maintain the dignity and self-esteem of a person who has been incontinent are at the heart of skilled practice. This exploration allowed me the opportunity to look at both the hidden world of nursing and expert practice in an 'invisible' area.

The next stage

The practitioners felt it important to keep field notes about their immediate feelings and thoughts when an interaction involving touch occurred. These would form *aides-mémoire* for them in their discussion with their clinical supervisors and aid debate in subsequent reflective practice groups. This reflects one of the problems of reflecting on practice. How do we do this without altering the experience through our memory? How well do diaries or short notes help to capture the essence of the experience? However, this is not the story of their experience but primarily of my own.

I decided to examine touch in a similar way. The reasons for this involve my general interest in the 'invisible' areas of practice, and a need I felt to see if I could gain insight into my own practice in the ways that the practitioners were exploring their practice. There I was facilitating the work of a group who were exploring practice and judgement in a particular way. It seemed a sensible approach but I needed to gain confidence and expertise for myself. To an extent, I may have felt it was wrong to persuade or nudge people down a path I had not tried.

Comment

It is important to note that this is not a formal study but an approach which grew out of, or evolved from, my working with a group of practitioners. However, in the world of practice this can be an effective approach to developing insights into and learning from our practice. It also provides insight into the practical problems for both practitioners and lecturers in this approach. Both groups have a whole variety of responsibilities, demands on time, and are subject to the pressures of getting today's work done. Creating space to think strategically, finding periods to examine practice and reflect on judgement can be difficult. Yet that world is a reality, and it is within it that we must create the windows or opportunities for this critical and vital work.

My own journey

In order to start this enquiry I had to negotiate time in a clinical area where I could examine and reflect on my own practice. It was a fascinating experience returning to partial involvement in clinical practice. Fascinating in terms of comparing and contrasting my usual involvement with practice, which was through being with practitioners, as opposed to being once more back in practice myself with real patients!

Normally I worked with practitioners in discussing and analysing their experience. One is in a position where one gets a vicarious immersion in practice. In again being more involved myself with people, the immediate feelings were of being rusty, slightly out of tune, off-key and clumsy. It was as if I knew the words to the part but the performance was wooden. The term professional mastery is being explored in literature and research. Perhaps we need to explore the term professional rustiness as well!

These feelings would bear out the literature that suggests 'expertise in nursing derives from familiarity with the "doing" of nursing and requires a practitioner to be fully immersed in practice' (Sutton and Smith, 1995, p. 1038). Involvement with practice and practitioners can help develop heightened understanding of expert practice but active engagement in sustained practice is necessary to maintain clinical expertise.

In discussing my experience there were several frameworks or approaches to reflecting on practice that could be used. These include those by Boud, Keogh and Walker (1985), Gibbs (1988), Mezirow (1981) and Johns (1995). Johns' approach, adapted from Carper's (1978) work on patterns of knowing, is perhaps the most widely used in the past few years.

Selecting an appropriate framework for thinking about practice is a potential problem. As the number of possible frameworks increase, which one is appropriate for one's own journey? Some of the approaches give the feel that thinking and reflection are 'either/or' phenomena, which means you are either a reflective practitioner or you are not. Van Manen (1990), however, makes the obvious but frequently overlooked point that reflection is not like this and that there are various levels of reflection. As Derbyshire argues, 'as human beings and as nurses we do think and reflect every day. We bring common-sense understandings to a myriad novel and familiar situations and interpret our world minute by minute as we experience it' (Derbyshire, 1993, p. 28).

Van Manen's approach to levels of thinking is intuitively attractive to me. This phenomenological approach proposes that there are several types of reflection: anticipatory reflection, active reflection, mindfulness and recollective reflection. It is this framework that will guide my discussion of my own practice.

Anticipatory reflection

This kind of thinking involves consideration of various approaches to a person's care, possible courses of action and intervention, the planning of care and anticipation of the effect and outcomes of intervention.

In caring for a variety of people during my periods in practice, I was conscious that, within their overall care, I was particularly interested in a specific range of interventions. This caused me some ethical and moral concerns. This was not an 'objective' or 'disembodied' process. I was actively involved in care. Would the care of the people I worked with be affected by this?

In addition to this feeling, in considering my possible interventions I was conscious of those raised by the practitioners in the reflective practice group. Would there be a danger I was testing out the forms of touch they had identified rather than exploring my own practice?

I also felt obliged, perhaps by my traditional academic background, to re-examine the literature on touch. This was superbly summarised by Bottorff (1991) in her methodological review and evaluation of research on nurse–patient touch. This examines twenty-seven unpublished and fifty-six published research projects. This was another dilemma. Would it have been better to have looked at the literature after re-immersing myself in practice or before? If this had been a research study the design would have helped clarify this choice.

The reason for my choice was the fact that if I was caring for people then I felt bound to consider whether or not my practice should be influenced by the evidence that already existed. In fact the literature helped very little. Touch within a nurse–patient relationship has been researched from a variety of perspectives. Definitions, description, measurement and evaluation of the effects, are all dimensions that had been examined. However, there was little on the form of touch that we were looking at, and virtually nothing on how we chose to respond to a patient touching us.

As Bottorff, concludes:

The review of the literature reinforces the fact that little is known with certainty about nurse–patient touch. The lack of definitive findings in this field is due to the influence of unsubstantiated a priori assumptions that underlie the predominantly deductive approaches used to investigate touch, the lack of attention to the context in which touch occurs (which is central to an understanding of touch), methodological problems, and problems associated with the definition of touch. (Bottorff, 1991, p. 338)

Comment

I was fascinated and appalled to realise the absence of research into the effect of patients touching us as health professionals. None of these eighty-three studies examined this fact. How much research is aimed at exploring what we do as health professionals, and does not adequately examine how a patient or client alters that behaviour? A relationship does involve more than one person. Perhaps the idea of a passive patient is more powerful than I thought!

It also made me realise that the traditional approach, of first examining the literature, does not always help. It did not provide me with cues as to my own practice in this area. This is a small example of the issue that met social science researchers who found that traditional research methodologies were unhelpful, and has led to the debate on new paradigm research.

How many times do we find that existing literature does not fit? Is that a primary cause of why we need to develop our professional judgement? We learn to rely on ourselves and our judgement where the problems of the people we care for, or teach, or meet in our own practice, do not fit the existing written knowledge.

So armed with my anxieties over how 'rusty' I would be, concerns for whether the care I would give would be appropriate for those for whom I was caring, and a failed attempt to relieve my anxieties by examining the literature, I spent a period in an appropriate practice setting.

Clinical experience

I arranged with the staff on an acute elderly mentally ill ward to spend three shifts a week for two weeks there. They wore uniforms in this area, so this involved searching a cupboard to find an old white coat that was presentable! So with a placement arranged, a white coat and a mixture of anticipation and anxiety I went to work.

A number of the qualified nurses on the ward were colleagues I taught on post-registration degree schemes at the university. The student nurses present were also known to me as they were on the undergraduate degree programme of which I was Course Leader! Not unexpectedly, my arrival was greeted with some cheerful banter.

Their reactions were fun. These ranged over: "Oh, so you are going to be a proper nurse again" or "it does mean getting your hands dirty" and "so you can experience the theory–practice gap and not just talk about it". They were supportive, but it reinforced for me the importance of academic staff in professional disciplines being involved in practice. The credibility of the messenger is undoubtedly enhanced.

In practical terms, my clinical experience involved supporting the caring of a group of people under the supervision of their primary nurse. We had nine clients in the shift for whom we were directly responsible. At the end of the shift, or if there was time during it, I wrote short notes of my experience in general and specific comments about critical incidents in relation to touch. In particular I tried to reflect, when responding to being touched, whether my professional judgement enabled me to know which need was to be met and therefore which interventions I should use.

So what did I learn? Returning to Van Manen's approach to thinking, what were my active thoughts?

Active reflection

This approach to thinking can be described as 'thinking on your feet', or keeping your wits about you, rather than working on auto pilot, and being aware of what you are doing as you do it. This is undoubtedly the most controversial area of reflective practice.

It is controversial because, reflecting in action, from a calculative or technical rational thinking perspective would involve practitioners standing back (metaphorically and possibly literally) from their practice in order to consider their actions. However, the real world of practice rarely allows for such reflective distancing in the midst of caring.

There is also a real danger, as Derbyshire states, that 'reflection in action could actually be detrimental to expert practice. For example, nursing is often described as an intimate and complex psychomotor and psycho-social caring practice.' He argues, 'if, rather like making love, we take this approach, this sort of thinking could actually lead to a breakdown of a smooth performance'. It is important to remember that, as Derbyshire says, 'in much of excellent nursing and teaching practice we have a non-reflective, intuitive grasp of what we are doing, which most assuredly does not mean that we are practising thoughtlessly' (Derbyshire, 1993, p. 28).

My own experience

This debate, which is critical in an understanding of practice, was evident in my own experience. In noting my interactions with people in relation to touch and how I responded, there was at first a tendency to 'detach' myself from the experience. I was thinking: "what am I doing and why did I choose to do that?" A comment from my own notes states: 'in pausing to think, it makes me feel clumsy and slow'. Perhaps this is a reflection of functioning nearer the novice practitioner end of Benner's (1992) continuum of advanced beginner – competent – proficient – expert.

Advanced beginners, Benner argues, use learned procedures to infer from the clinical situation the immediate requirements for action. This contrasts with expert practitioners who recognise patterns and grasp situations immediately and directly. I was having to think consciously about my judgement in relation to touch. It felt like being out of tune or slightly off-key. The artistry was hampered by deliberation. My judgement appeared to be based on a degree of trial and error.

This was classically shown by my reaction when a person did 'clutch' me. They were unable to communicate verbally but were agitated and distressed. I responded purely to the behaviour. I did not yet know the person or have a feel for them. So I ended up testing out whether they wanted a drink, to go to the lavatory, be held, or needed to be anchored to me for a period.

My judgement was slow and I was forced to run through a series of options. Perhaps in this case it may seem this was not crucial to the person's care. In a life-threatening situation this delay may have caused serious problems. However, for this person it did mean that they were in a state of distress for longer than they should have been. As the aim of the care was to alleviate distress then this level of expertise did not help the person as quickly as it should have done.

As my time in practice increased, this feeling changed. My judgement became proficient. I felt in tune with the people for whom I cared. Although this is reflected in my notes, I was now recording these at the end of a period of working. So perhaps it can be argued, this is not 'true' reflection in action. However, it bore out for me how difficult it is to reflect in action without disturbing the harmony between oneself and the person for whom one is caring. It felt, for me, as though this harmony was the backcloth to exercising professional judgement.

As Benner *et al.* state: 'Central to the clinical judgement of expert nurses is what they describe in their every day discourse as "knowing the patient", this means both knowing the patient's typical patterns of responses and knowing the patient as a person' (Benner *et al.* 1996, p. 20). The harmony I began to feel was certainly related to feeling I was starting to know the people for whom I was caring. This was demonstrated to me by the awareness that I was responding more smoothly and accurately to being touched. I was developing a 'feel' as to which need the person wanted meeting. My judgement was improving.

These thoughts about harmony are more related to the area of reflection that Van Manen calls mindfulness. It illustrates the problem of perhaps trying to make one's reflective thoughts fit a model or approach. Instead, with hindsight, it may be more helpful to free oneself of these approaches and trust one's own judgement about the way to reflect on professional practice!

Mindfulness

Mindfulness and thoughtfulness are ways of being involved thoughtfully in situations where we are 'actively and immediately involved in a manner of consciousness that only later is open to true reflection' (Van Manen, 1991, p. 123). This level of thinking generated feelings which were developed from the concept of harmony. Skilled practice is a performance. An actor, a dancer or a painter must rehearse or practise. Their judgement about a nuance, or an expression, or a blend of colour, is a result of hours of practice. It is within that context that those practitioners make a judgement.

The similarities between a skilled performance by a dancer and by a nurse, in terms of artistry of performance, are well argued by Picard (1995). Excellent care-based nursing requires an inner-centredness and harmony like a dancer or like an artist. Nightingale wrote:

> Nursing is an art but if it is to be an art, it requires as exclusive a devotion and as hard a preparation as any painter's or sculptor's work; for what is having to do with dead canvas or cold marble compared with having to do with the living body, the temple of God's spirit? (Tooley, 1910, p. 123)

This feeling that a skilled performance is related to hard preparation was borne out by my own experience. The final shift of work I engaged in was smoother and more skilled in terms of my practice. The other shifts had been rehearsals for the final performance! The problem in health care or education is that these rehearsals take place with patients or students.

In the desire for evidence-based practice, or clinical effectiveness, or research-based practice, how much of the skills of professional judgement will remain misunderstood if we neglect our understanding of the artistry of skilled or expert practice?

Recollective reflection

This involves consideration of the success of practices and interventions. We can take time to contemplate the deeper meanings of our practices and to uncover what they tell us about being a nurse and giving care.

In undertaking this level of thinking I worked with the mental health reflective group to share our experiences. This felt different from previous meetings for me. In other discussions I had had a primary role in facilitating their understanding of their practice. In this group it was my practice as well as their own that we were exploring.

The themes that emerged from sharing and analysing our experience were refinements of those discussed earlier that emerged from the previous reflective group that had examined touch. The same forms of intervention were identified. However, what had become clearer to us, was the basis on which the judgement was made, as to which intervention to use. This judgement was clearly based on feeling how well we 'knew' the person and how we intuitively 'felt their need'. We articulated how, in caring for people for whom words as a means of communication may be inadequate, we had developed an understanding of how the people we cared for displayed 'agitation' or 'restlessness' or 'distress' or 'unease' or 'contentment'. This was shown through the person's whole self, the 'way they were'.

Is this not similar to an artist who may have developed the expertise to know what shade of a particular colour to use? Is judgement, for both the artist and the expert practitioner, not then inextricably bound up with the artistry of practice? The conviction that 'something is not right', or 'the picture doesn't feel right', or a person is 'going off', are perhaps expressions of expertly developed practice.

Perhaps this illustrates the complexities of exercising judgement. Is exercising one particular judgement enmeshed and entangled with our overall judgement or 'feel' for a person? Does the world of objective evidence, outcome measures, random controlled trials, simply shrug its shoulders at such messy, unquantifiable work?

Although there is an increasing body of work examining this form of approach, which it is not within the scope of this chapter to explore, considerably more work is still required to understand the complexities of exercising judgement.

Finally, this level of thinking also encourages people to explore the deeper meanings of their practice. This certainly happened in relation to debating this form of touch. It led, for me, to questioning a whole range of issues. These included: the whole philosophy underpinning the care of people with this range of problems; the aims of care; the direction of health care in relation to people who require care rather than cure as their central need; how we develop trustful relationships; how we show connectedness and the use of our presence; and how we argue to keep skilled practitioners in this field of practice when it may appear to be an area suitable to unskilled practitioners. How did we, in fact, articulate expert practice and the skilled use of judgement?

These debates, conducted in subsequent groups, were stimulating and it did show how concentrating on one area of practice generates new enthusiasm, ideas and insights into the whole nature of professional practice.

Concluding thoughts

The overriding thought is that understanding the use of professional judgement is complex. It involves exploring the artistry of skilled practice, and such artistry can be hard to define. But in a world at present tilted towards measurable outcomes, standards, targets, meta-analyses and effectiveness, as Van Manen argues, 'the teachers' ability and inclination to reflect thoughtfully on the pedagogical nature of their lives with students are being atrophied by the objectifying and alienating conditions under which they work' (Van Manen, 1990, p. 321).

However, this work remains, I am convinced, of critical importance. The measurable evidence of practice is small. Expert clinical practice is like an iceberg, with one tenth on show (identifiable evidence) and nine tenths below the surface (artistry). Yet, the hidden and invisible world 'below', may well be what governs how, and whether, evidence is used.

The challenge facing us, is to make this expert practice explicit, and to show that it cannot be standardised. It will vary in its use from one person to another, and from one context to another. Academic and clinical colleagues readily accept thinking that acknowledges the beauty of a picture, or the expertness of a performance by a dancer or actor. We must strive to transfer the acceptance of this approach to thinking in relation to art and music, into the world of expert practice and the exercising of professional judgement.

References

Benner, P. (1984). *From Novice to Expert: Excellence and Power in Clinical Nursing Practice*. Addison-Wesley.

Benner, P., Tanner, C. and Chesla, C. (1992). From beginner to expert: gaining a differentiated clinical world in critical care nursing. *Advances in Nursing Science*, **14**, 13–28.

Benner, P., Tanner, C. and Chesla, C. (1996). *Expertise in Nursing Practice: Caring, Clinical Judgement and Ethics.* Springer.

Bottorff, J. (1991). A methodological review and evaluation of research on nurse–patient touch. In *Anthology on Caring* (P. Chinn, ed.), pp. 321–334. National League for Nursing Press.

Boud, D., Keogh, R. and Walker, D. (1985). *Reflection: Turning Experience into Learning.* Kogan Page.

Carper, B. (1978). Fundamental ways of knowing in nursing. *Advances in Nursing Science,* 1, 13–23.

Clarke, M. (1986). Action and reflection: practice and theory in nursing. *Journal of Advanced Nursing,* 11, 3–11.

Derbyshire, P. (1993). In the halls of mirrors. *Nursing Times,* 8 December, pp. 26–29.

Gibbs, G. (1988). *Learning by Doing. A Guide to Teaching and Learning Methods.* Further Education Unit, Oxford Polytechnic.

Graham, I. (1996). A presentation of a conceptual framework and its use in the definition of nursing development within a number of nursing development units. *Journal of Advanced Nursing,* 23, 260–266.

Greenwood, J. (1993). Reflective practice: a critique of the work of Argyris and Schön. *Journal of Advanced Nursing,* 18, 1183–1187.

Johns, C. (1995). Framing learning through reflection within Carper's fundamental ways of knowing in nursing. *Journal of Advanced Nursing,* 22, 226–234.

Kottkamp, R. (1990). Means for facilitating reflection. *Education and Urban Society,* 22, 182–203.

Lawler, J. (1991). *Behind the Screens: Nursing, Somology, and the Problem of the Body.* Churchill Livingstone.

Lumby, J. (1991). *Nursing: Reflecting on an Evolving Practice.* Deakin University Press.

Mezirow, J. (1981). A critical theory of adult learning and education. *Adult Education,* 32, 3–24.

Picard, C. (1995). Caring in nursing and dance. *Journal of Holistic Nursing,* 13, 323–331.

Powell, J. (1989). The reflective practitioner in nursing. *Journal of Advanced Nursing,* 14, 824–832.

Reed, J. and Proctor, S. (1993). *Nurse Education: A Reflective Approach.* Edward Arnold.

Schön, D. A. (1983). *The Reflective Practitioner.* Basic Books.

Street, A. (1991). *From Image to Action: Reflection in Nursing Practice.* Deakin University Press.

Sutton, S. and Smith, C. (1995). Advanced nursing practice: new ideas and new perspectives. *Journal of Advanced Nursing,* 21, 1037–1043.

Tooley, S. (1910). *The Life of Florence Nightingale.* Cassell.

Van Manen, M. (1990). *Researching Lived Experience: Human Science for an Action-Sensitive Pedagogy.* Althouse Press.

Van Manen, M. (1991). *The Tact of Teaching: the Meaning of Pedagogical Thoughtfulness.* State University of New York Press.

Weiss, S. J. (1979). The language of touch. *Nursing Research,* 28, 76–80.

Part Three

Responding to Practice as Artistry

Della Fish and Colin Coles

Chapter 11

From reflection to critical appreciation: learning to respond to the artistry of practice

Introduction

The contributors have each provided in Part Two a case study based upon detailed reflections on an incident from their practice. These case studies can be placed on a continuum from descriptive through interpretative to highly deliberative. All go beyond offering an uncritical narrative of events and entail critical reflections on and theorising about their practice, and all recognise that even apparently simple narrative would contain interpretation. Most go further than this and grapple in detail with the complexities of practice which they characterise as contestable and problematic and raise for themselves and the reader issues about which there is need for deeper deliberation, and which the reader too sees as matters for serious thought.

Where each chapter lies on the continuum from descriptive to deliberative case study depends upon how far, in addition to theorising his or her own practice, each writer has drawn upon the perspectives of others, tapped into key professional problems and used formal theory in order to relate their individual practice to wider issues. (We contrast this use of theory with other justifiable uses where, for example, practitioners refer to it in order to support, express better, or extend their own ideas, and/or to demonstrate their credentials as members of a scholarly community, or less justifiable ones, for example, for the sake of conforming to convention in writing, where theory is used to no real end.)

All the chapters in Part Two then offer examples of what can be achieved in case study, employing reflection on and deliberation about professional practice. But, we would argue, this important understanding of practice can be taken a step further. That is, we believe that it is also highly instructive, for those who subscribe to the professional artistry view of their work, to respond to that very artistry and also to consider the artistry involved in the written presentation of that practice. In order to illustrate what we mean by this, we offer in Part Three our own appreciation of our contributors' work and their writing, as an example of how a practitioner might look at his or her own practice. Further details about appreciating the artistry of practice can also be found in Fish (in press).

Part Three as a whole then, attempts to offer the various elements which constitute a critical appreciation of the collection of our contributors' writing. First we offer in this chapter some introductory information about critical appreciation and explain how we set about this work, together with some matters which provide a context for understanding further the writing under study. In the following chapter we provide our main response to the voices of our writers. The third and final chapter of this section focuses on professional judgement which is singled out for attention because it lies at the core of our contributors' work and is the central focus of this publication.

Initial overview

The writers of the previous six chapters have allowed us to hear their voices as practitioners who are struggling to understand and make sense of incidents from their individual practice and link them to the traditions of the practices of their profession. What they reveal are processes of thinking in all (or many) of its layers and not simply the end products of their reflections. This means that although they may have begun their thinking by locating a vivid incident which crystallises their dilemmas, in writing about this they are doing far more than simply telling a story – they are simultaneously telling it and investigating it and sharing with us the fits and starts in their voyages of understanding. This means that the structure of their work portrays in some way the 'messy' nature of their professional practice, the trials and errors of their investigative process and the undulating path of their understanding. Because they have captured and reflected upon the processes of their own thinking and acting, their narratives often lurch unpredictably between insight and mystification, and certainty and insecurity. This in itself opens up professional practice in health care to the recognition of important but often previously cloaked professional problems. What they do not provide and what we now seek to offer is a slightly more distanced view of their practice which seeks to respond to its artistry and the art of their writing.

Readers who already engage in the process of reflecting on their practice will know that in many cases it really is exactly as portrayed in T. S. Eliot's famous words:

> We shall not cease from exploration
> And the end of all our exploring
> Will be to arrive where we started
> And know the place for the first time.

> ('Little Gidding', V: 26–29)

For this reason we, as readers, may hear these contributors saying in one sentence things that are apparently simple, obvious and seemingly trivial and that we already feel we know, and yet in the very next words hear them offering from out of their private and intimate crises insights new to writer and reader, or some illumination which staggers, excites, teases, or worries. We argue that this of itself should alert us to the need to read this work more deeply. The whole of Part Three is offered as an example of such 'reading' – in all its facets.

Intentions of Part Three: the task of critical appreciation

The ultimate intention of this book is to free readers to conduct their own explorations of their own practice and thus to see the examples offered in the previous six chapters as well as in this and the next two chapters, not as new knowledge to be applied to their own practice but simply as examples of reflection on practice and appreciation of it, aimed at encouraging them to conduct similar yet different explorations into their own practice. There is a need, however, in the intermediate term to understand these cases – even if only to extend our appreciation of professional practice and its traditions. To this end we offer our 'reading' of these contributions, taking account of the complexity of their professional work and of its portrayal on paper and with due recognition that we have been privileged to look at moments in the development of colleagues' understanding.

At one level, what we offer here is simply *our* response to the previous six chapters, and we hope (and strongly urge) that as a result of it, readers will, before turning to Part Four, be drawn to re-read the contributor's work, in order to see what they themselves now make of it in the light of our views. Indeed, such reiteration, constantly oscillating between practice and theory, is an underlying theme in this book as it is of professional development.

At another level, however, what we offer here is fundamentally different from what is usually produced in response to case studies or other kinds of humanistic research. And in that sense we are also offering a model of what we mean by critical appreciation.

The '*processing*' of case studies usually provides what a researcher is often at pains to argue is an unequivocal analysis of the case (atomising it into categories, producing numerical data, weighing up the significance of the components and, as a result, arguing strongly for a particular interpretation of the data 'captured' and 'created' within the research). Such a reading of the data (as opposed to reading the case) is almost always interested in separating out the parts from the whole – what might be characterised as 'reading into it rather than reading it'. The resulting analysis is then usually extrapolated across the cases by seeking to emphasise common categories in order to present an overwhelming argument for the conclusions of the research. This of course is useful where new scientific knowledge is being sought and tested. It seems to us less relevant where understanding some aspect of the human condition is the ultimate aim, and where it is important in that cause to do justice to the unity or wholeness of the writing. In that case, readers need to see in it, and as endemic to it, the elements that have been separated out, and even then should see them only as *part* of its overall nature, some elements of art being essentially ineffable or unable to be fully articulated except indirectly in images or shadows.

Thus our research is not aimed at producing final conclusions, and as a result offering new information to be applied by practitioners during their daily work. Rather it is concerned with making, in company with colleagues, an inner journey, a voyage in which action and its subterranean counterpart, thought, are explored. In this sense, our contributors' writing is more like art (which often seeks to shape and offer action and uncover thought for the audience's appreciation), and our response is more like art criticism in that it employs the *art* of appreciation. Thus we are concerned with understanding the complexities of professional practice by means of the processes of responding to the understandings of others. This can only be done with integrity if each case is viewed and considered *as a whole* rather than in some atomised form, and, further, if the collection of cases itself is similarly apprehended as a unity.

Examples of this idea of a collection within which each piece of art both stands alone and contributes to a new whole might be found in most of the arts. At one level it can be found where someone other than the artist has brought a collection together which then makes new meanings beyond those found in the individual items collected (for example in an art gallery or museum, where an exhibition has been put together which focuses on the work of an artist or on a theme or topic). It can also be found in the deliberate collection *by the artist* of individual pieces to make a unity which is offered to the public. Examples might include Sir Philip Sidney's famous collection of 108 sonnets and eleven songs called *Astrophel and Stella* (from which we quote below), John Donne's sonnet sequence 'La Corona', and even perhaps T. S. Eliot's *Old Possum's Book of Practical Cats* (though whether the musical *Cats* is a modern dance example which achieves the same unity is a moot point). Certainly, examples are not confined to literature. Mussorgsky's *Pictures at an Exhibition*, and the dance sequence based on the work of Lowry and designed for television, also come to mind.

Perhaps, however, the supreme example of this is to be found in literature, in James Joyce's collection of short stories called *Dubliners*. Here each story is a gem in itself and even in isolation from the rest offers up riches to the reader who will stop to discern the voice, the character and the moral stance of the Dubliner around whom that story is focused. Taken together, however, the whole fifteen short stories offer a variety of voices from the city of Dublin which then constitute a unity which Joyce himself referred to as 'a chapter in the moral history of my country'.

Critical appreciation, critical analysis and critical interpretation

In a properly critical and responsive reading of *Dubliners* it would do no justice to the sensibilities there portrayed to count how many times in one chapter or even in the collection as a whole there occurs a particular image (like the fog, which is clearly used as a symbol of the moral paralysis of that city). Such critical *analysis*, with its penchant for quantification, is often written in response to art, but we would argue that a critical appreciation is something different. We would also distinguish it from a critical *interpretation*, which might impose upon the original meaning and intentions of the author some vision which is demonstrably more the critic's than the writer's. Thus, as is clear from *Dubliners* itself, and as an appreciation of it would also make clear, the reader is intended to recognise the apparent ubiquitousness of the 'murky air', and discern from its place in the whole, the clear meaning of this image and its significance in the overall picture being painted and under-lying morals being probed. It is to these and not to the quanti-fication of the image or the artifice of his or her own interpretation that the critic providing an *appreciation* of the work would draw readers' attention.

We would argue that there is a parallel between these responses to literature (or other art) and responses to educational research of all kinds. Research reports or studies in the positivistic or scientific paradigm offer matters which will yield to analysis, those in the humanistic paradigm offer a range of interpretations. Each of these seeks a similar response from a reader. By contrast, case studies which are essentially about the artistry of practice deserve to be responded to through critical appreciation.

We thus seek to share our response – our critical appreciation – of each of the chapters above and the unity they together constitute, in order to help readers to discern what these writers (and we as educators) believe is worth taking seriously in this work. For this purpose we abandon the role of editor in this section of the book and adopt the role of art critic, seeking to recognise what is being said in all its subtlety about professional practice and to consider the significance of, and to highlight, some of the means by which it is being said and to recognise the distinguishing qualities of the writing.

Eisner usefully defines the term 'appreciation' in the context of critical appreciation as 'an awareness and an understanding of what one has experienced which provides a basis for judgement' and as being quite neutral about 'liking' the object of such attention. He then says that such critical appreciation is *'the art of disclosure'*, in that it renders vivid the qualities of the subject under scrutiny. He is at pains to define it as doing more than awakening sensibility, but rather as demonstrating the subject's history, social context and tradition and how they depart from the conventional (Eisner, 1985, p. 105). It might thus be said that the role of such a critic is to enlighten the reader's response to a piece of art by offering significant contextual information about it, and then pointing to and thus indicating what he or she sees in it, in order to help others to see something too. And because something pointed out involves a pointer and an observer, this image alerts us to the significance of the two parties to this transaction: the person (or persona) pointing and the 'pointer's' audience. As well as working faithfully on the text under study, the critic must also provide a clear indication of the basis of his or her work and establish a relationship with the reader (as we now seek to do). Then, just as our contributors have come to see their practice in a new light, so we as critics need first to recognise and then to enable our readers to see that writing anew – even to see beyond or beneath what the writers themselves have articulated. It will then be for the audience (of the original case studies and of our appreciation of them) to decide on their own response to both, which we would hope would be neither to accept nor reject our writing but to explore it and extend further their own understandings).

The intentions of our critical appreciation (or critical commentary) of the previous six chapters then are as follows.

1 To respond – as active and discerning readers who are also reflective practitioners – to the printed word and through that to the ideas it enshrines about professional practice, to the wholeness of the individual chapters and the unity that they

constitute (the integrity, harmony, balance, proportion and symmetry).

2 Whilst so doing, to give evidence of our reliability as honest and diligent critics, to treat the writers and their work with a proper respect and attend to the relationship which we develop with our (and their) readers.

3 To point to and thus to point out (indicate) the qualities of the writing, to nudge the reader to see links and patterns, and locate, recognise and probe the insights. This involves:

- providing such contextual matters as are necessary to appreciate the work
- seeing and highlighting what each writer is trying to do and say (such intentions, as well as being stated can, as we shall see, be reached through imagery, tone, mood, style)
- getting behind the surface of the words to what may be being said at a deeper level
- pointing up the writers' attitudes to their subject
- making an effort to understand how the writers *present* their work
- recognising the themes and ideas being explored and to think about their significance
- highlighting the writers' sensibilities by drawing attention to nuance, mood and tone as well as imagery and style
- considering how form and structure themselves convey, support and even elaborate upon content
- looking at pattern and balance, continuity and development
- considering the moral content as it emerges via style, tone and mood, and through the stated and the implied values, beliefs and assumptions
- identifying and celebrating the spirit which shines through it
- seeing how the reader's judgements are brought about.

It should be noted too that the critical appreciation of a subject can be illuminated by reference to and comparison with some other art form or another example of the same form. (For example, considering two poems on the same topic often enables a reader to say more about each than would be possible in meeting them alone.) In some cases even, the writer or maker deliberately sets up such comparisons and references. And since art is often a means of crystallising some aspect of real life to be explored in detail by artist and public, there is no reason why relevant art should not be used to illuminate by comparison professional research which is seeking to crystallise and explore elements of professional practice. That is what we are doing below as we elaborate upon the parallels between this work and *Dubliners*. Such comparisons only occurred to us after we looked at the completed collection in Part Two; our writers only heard about them after this chapter had been written, at which point it transpired that none had ever read Joyce's work.

To be sure, we do not wish to imply a greater significance in the work of our contributors than they do themselves. Certainly, too, some chapters show greater moral seriousness than others, but all the contributing writers are alert to the significance of some aspects of their practice, and in this we can learn from them about our relationship to our own. Further, their professional practice is itself, as we have already argued, characterisable as artistry, and their writing about it has been deliberately shaped and controlled according to some of the principles of art (which were shared in a workshop towards the end of the time they spent writing). Art can be defined as something original, 'well made', with a relationship to a tradition of 'making' and whose high qualities deserve to be recognised. We aim, then, to help readers to discern what the contributors want us to take seriously, to respond to it as a whole and to recognise the artistry in it.

It will be noted from this that we seek to avoid the abuse of criticism so often evident when the critic tries to make of or impose upon his or her subject, those meanings, intentions and concerns for which there is no evidence. We seek to respond to what the writers are seeking to say. Although what we offer is still our interpretation, we have tried to ensure that it responds to what is in the writing, by referencing our comments back to the original text, thus leaving the reader to decide ultimately on the value of our comments. We have also taken the precaution of sharing and checking out our responses with our writers.

The processes involved in our initial appreciation

The basis of our own response to the writings presented in Part Two is a very careful reading, which attended to the writers' intentions as discernible from the writing, to the detail of meanings in each chapter and to how they are conveyed. We therefore read through the entire set of chapters, responding to them holistically, and then re-read them. We noted carefully during both readings what we believed the writers to be saying, making various checks against the text and sharing our perceptions of this. We came to all this open-mindedly. We also noted how the form and style underlined the content, by means of the shape and form of the piece, the judicious selection of vocabulary, the texture of language (style) and tone of voice. During our second reading we marked their text at any and all points where we noted something of significance. These markings we then transferred to index cards and sought amongst them common themes, forms and styles and how these related to the writers' original intentions (and with awareness of our own as editors). From these we shaped the chapter which follows this.

The contributors' intentions

The discerned intentions of our writers then are proper starting and finishing points for a critical appreciation of their writing. In this case we mean their detailed as well as their overall intentions, some of which they themselves only discovered during the course of their writing. We shall try to come at these by probing further the comparison made above between the work of our contributors and that of Joyce's *Dubliners*.

This comparison is defensible at a number of levels. We are not, of course, making any claim that the quality of writing as art is at the level of Joyce's. This would be foolish since our contributors do not aspire to be great literary writers. Their artistry is of another kind, and certainly lacks the economy of style that is the hallmark of Joyce's work in *Dubliners*. The comparison is none the less relevant because Joyce on the one hand and our writers on the other offer us as readers a series of portraits which are successful both at the level of individual chapters and as a unified collection. Further, each offers voices and characters through whom we learn about some serious matters of life. We know that *Dubliners* was designed to offer us events in a moral drama via the intimate crises of each character round whom a chapter is written. (There is published critique suggesting that each of the chapters explores one particular vice through the characters and actions portrayed, see Ghiselin, 1956.) How sustainable this idea is in detail is a matter of judgement focused on the text. What is indisputable, however, since he himself writes about them, are Joyce's moral intentions for the work. In a similar way our writers offer critical incidents in their practice which carry moral significance and are understood by writers and readers by means of the writers' reflections upon them. *Dubliners*, being a work of prose fiction, is ultimately about manners and morals and provides a commentary on the impoverished spiritual state that was Dublin's malaise in the early 1900s (the book being written between 1904 and 1908 and published in 1914). Through material focused upon their *real* professional practice, our contributors offer insights – across five professions – into their agonising and uncertainties and show us the malaise of spirit which currently characterises their professional working situations. This all vividly demonstrates the dilemmas associated, for those who work in health care, with taking moral responsibility and exercising professional judgement in a climate where there is much talk of ethics but where moral subtleties are often neither valued nor even recognised and where other values – those of the market place – are in the ascendant. And what they have to say is all the more significant because it is written by well-established and senior members of their professions.

Further, *Dubliners* starts in autobiographical form, its first three stories being told from that viewpoint. It then opens out into third person narrative and the past tense as the later stories begin to reveal more overtly the nature of the public world of Dublin that lies behind the individual characters. Similarly, our writers (at least in practice if not in the final form of their writing) began by attempting to capture and understand an occurrence (an intimate drama) in their professional life, which opened out into recounting some more personal aspects of their own living (their search first for meanings and then for evidence and their exploring of connections), and which finally saw them demonstrating how the personal and the professional is inextricably related and how as a result of looking carefully at their individual and more private practice they are compelled to raise major and profound questions about wider and more public matters. And there is ample evidence of this. Rosemary, for example, talks of how we define situations from our own experience, our own biography, how we are influenced in our understanding of our practice by the moral, ethical and ideological position we (often unconsciously) occupy at the time and she then comes to consider the influence on practice of its social context.

Thus, by drawing parallels between the work of our contributors and of *Dubliners*, we can come to see these portraits of practitioners as more than a simple series of sketches of professional practice but rather as a series of chapters in the moral history of and the present spiritual condition of professional practice in health care.

As we shall see, the agonising they illustrate, which is endemic to the exercising of both professional action and moral responsibilities, aptly demonstrates the desperate need in professional development to nourish, support and educate professional judgement.

Contextual matters

Autobiographical form: its historical context

The work of our contributors, then, is firmly in the tradition of autobiographical writing, about which much has already been written of its contribution to reflective research and its uses in humanistic enquiry (for example: Abbs; Boud, Keogh and Walker; Grumet; Pinar, and Woods). Perhaps less, however, has been done in professional literature to remember that autobiography was first of all an art form in itself, whose roots may be traced back deep into the history of literary studies. It is instructive to pursue these matters briefly even if only to set autobiography in its richer context and be more fully aware of the traditions in which our contributors' work may be understood.

Although there were 'historiographers' before the days of Elizabeth the First, biography (the presentation of an individual 'Life') was an underdeveloped form in Tudor England. Indeed, the very word 'biography' did not become current before the 1680s. However, the genre established its hold in the seventeenth century with the work of Izaak Walton whose *Lives* (one of which was first published in 1640) recorded for the first time an interest in the minute details of ordinary life, and John Aubrey, who in *Brief Lives* (most of which was written between 1679 and 1680) revelled in its gossip. It was continued through Dryden, Boswell, Johnson and

Coleridge. Autobiography too, as a literary form, was established in England in the seventeenth century, and was becoming recognised as a literary genre by the 1660s. Indeed, that century favoured and fostered introspection, as no previous epoch in our history had done.

The first autobiography in English was written by a woman and belongs to the close of the Middle Ages. *The Book of Margery Kempe* in fact had rather more affinities with the confessional lives of the saints, but she also had an ear for worldly things and an observant eye, leaving a remarkable record of life and travel in the early fifteenth century.

The tide of interest in autobiographical writing was probably beginning to flow at the time when the poet Sidney wrote in the 1570s (in the famous words from the first sonnet of *Astrophel and Stella*): 'Look in thy heart and write'. (It is interesting to note that this phrase was remarkably closely echoed by Rosemary's: 'perhaps it is better to write from the heart than the head'). In fact Sidney still continued in the rest of that collection to write from inside the Petrarchan convention of courtly lover to distant lady. Not long afterwards, however, the work of John Donne played with and broke out of this stereotype and showed a strongly developed impulse for personal and vivid autobiography.

Indeed, the autobiographical impulse to crystallise the individual personal experience emerged at this time in poetry, plays, fiction and other forms of prose, including sermons and pamphlets, as well as other forms of art, including portraiture. It came to flower in seventeenth century England probably because the twin pressures of Humanism and Puritanism both urged upon people the extreme importance of taking individual responsibility, and the stirrings of democratic and egalitarian sentiments gave an impetus to chroniclers of ordinary lives. As Bottrall says, 'autobiography received great stimulus in Western Europe as a result of the Renaissance when the focus of men's interests shifted from eternity to time, and from the community to the individual' (Bottrall, 1958, p. 162). This period is also notable for the diaries and journals that were written – for example, the work of Pepys and Evelyn – which act even today as documents which record private experiences and responses to public events, and which are a rich resource for both humanistic and artistic enquiry. It is perhaps significant for our own purposes to recognise that when we read any such autobiography we are juggling with several perspectives at once – the writer's original and immediate view of events, thoughts and feelings (including sometimes that writer's sense of how posterity might judge him or her), the reader's modern response to all this and, mixed up with it, the view the modern reader gains through the advantage of hindsight which by definition was not available to the writer.

By the 1700s there were (and still are) two clear types of autobiography: the public memoir (the life story based on verifiable fact) which approximates to biography and is written for the benefit of contemporaries and posterity; and the rather more intimate autobiography based on self-scrutiny. Here authors are trying to explain why they are the kind of person they have turned out to be and why they think or behave in certain ways. Such a writer then, is concerned with self-knowledge and has affinities with the philosopher, poet and penitent. Here the interest is on the inner life and outward happenings are relegated to the background. The emphasis is on the spiritual and broadly educational development and the work is written for readers who find value in the thoughtfulness of their fellows.

As Margaret Bottrall points out, whilst 'memoirs' soon acquire a period flavour, self-analytical autobiography is less affected by time. As she says of this genre, 'Intuitive and emotional ways of reacting to experience do not alter much, although intellectual attitudes do' (Bottrall, 1958, p. 4). She puts this down to the fact that while we can recognise our own moods portrayed even in the literature of the ancient Hebrews and Greeks, nevertheless 'true self-knowledge is as elusive as ever it was'. She also adds:

> The intelligence that watches and comments is not separated from the self which is being watched. Nor is the self static; even in memory it has chameleon qualities. (Bottrall, 1958, p. 4)

She also neatly distinguishes the diary from the autobiography with the words:

> What principally differentiates [them] is the element of reconsideration. Both provide first hand evidence of life lived, and it may happen that the less pre-meditated record is truer to acts than the planned review. [But autobiography] is usually written from the vantage point that allows a wider survey and a much more deliberate choice of the episodes to be emphasised. There is consequently greater scope for self-deception, and for that slight degree of

falsification which so often accompanies the ordering of material for literary effect. (Bottrall, 1958, p. 5)

There is also scope, however, for thinking about the events, and for recognising in the apparently commonplace and trivial, their significant values, beliefs and assumptions. And there is room for conveying this more subtly and thus more meaningfully. Here, art can do what perhaps art is best at, namely offer intimations of the ineffable, reverberations of thoughts and ideas just beyond our grasp or our ability to articulate, or even face or name.

By contrast to this, some argue that there was growing a sense that people's 'real' life was more interesting than the life of the spirit, and that the idea that a person's private actions may be interesting to others may owe something to the spirit of scientific detachment which developed after the Renaissance. And here we have the beginnings of the tussle between objectivity and subjectivity, the arguments about which so haunt our contributors and so bedevil our own age – and not least the lives of researchers! For example, the unquestioned modern assumptions about the need for objectivity and positivism are visible in the half sense of guilt with which our contributors describe the strongly felt influence of the affective aspects of their professional lives. But the affective aspects have, of course, to be kept in balance with all the rest. And as we shall see below, Joyce, in his autobiographical novel *Portrait of the Artist as a Young Man,* has some very useful comments to make on the proper control of these elements. Further, for the writer of published autobiography, the one motivation explicitly to be *excluded* if the work is to be seen of some literary merit is that of writing *purely* for personal therapy. And all this in turn raises questions about the structure and form or shape of the narratives themselves, which literary studies can also help us to understand.

But, if these are the motivations for the writer, they also affect the reader. Why do people read autobiographies? Bottrall suggests one simple reason is 'to widen the boundaries of our own personal experience of people'. She adds: 'We may want to compensate for our own restrictions of daily life, or to reassure ourselves of our own normality ... no matter how many friends we may possess, no matter how far we may have travelled, we still need to supplement what we have learned at first hand. ... As we read them we lose and find ourselves; we are enlightened, entertained and liberated from the narrow confines of time, place and circumstance' (Bottrall, 1958, pp. 163–164). And this surely holds as true for the twentieth century professional reader of professional literature as for readers of literature through all the centuries.

In the light of all this, too, it is hardly surprising to learn that when the realistic novel sought greater realism and more social and psychological detail, it turned to autobiography – to the first person point of view as a way of enabling the reader to appreciate the complexity of life. And it is also relevant that the almost inevitable theme of a novel in which the story is told in the first person is the formation of that character, the motivation behind action, the complexity of thought and action and the apprenticeship or education of the main hero or heroine. It is from such novels that we learn how nuances can be contrived and enlightenment can be shed on the material provided through the autobiographical point of view by presenting chronological events in a different non-chronological order, by juxtaposing information, thought and action, by revealing a mismatch between the writer's views and his action, and by implying a discordance between the values enshrined in stated beliefs and those underlying self-presentation. We have, too, been brought face to face, through the modern novel and poetry, with the impossibility of coming to a simple ending when the material is autobiographical. Indeed, the end of an auto-biography can only be recorded by someone else – in a biography!

Autobiography as research

The six chapters in Part Two provide us with critical incidents in the practice of professionals. They are autobiographical. In chrono-logical terms the writers began their work by identifying and capturing on paper a critical incident from their own practice. This is now a very common approach to 'starting off' a piece of practitioner research. However, the similarities between their work and most previous practitioner research in health care begin and end with the identification of and the first sketching out of the incident.

What usually happens next (to caricature it slightly) is that the researchers formulate a research design and then act upon it. This is based on the idea (endemic in all positivist research) that it is important to rush off to 'investigate' further – by means of empirical work. Almost exclusively this has come to be seen to indicate two main activities. It involves burying oneself in professional writing (searching the literature) for answers to half formulated questions about what other people who have had similar experiences have thought, discovered and done. At the same time as this, or immediately afterwards, it involves the ritual of collecting or creating new data about one's practice. The nature of all such research designs is that action must be taken (and be seen to be taken) at considerable speed (and often to a tight deadline set before the work begins and almost inevitably too tight to do justice to the complexity that is uncovered later). This means coming to the arena of practice with an already narrowed (and particular) focus – one often set before practice has been in any way scrutinised, and certainly before any of its complexities have been revealed. When these researchers are full of matters which have taken them away from their real practice (to search for literature about other people's ideas and collect snippets of information about their own actions – inadequately contextualised and thus distorted and simplified) they then process the data in an attempt to come to some firm and preferably practical conclusions. And when it is all written up, the critical incident figures briefly, usually somewhere near the beginning. Ironically, it is only after all this has been completed that their real practice reappears on the agenda – as something to be got on with now the research is over!

By contrast, what our contributors (as researchers) do is to resist firmly the notion of rushing away from their autobiographies. Instead they reflect deeply upon them, treating *them* as their data for the purpose of all investigation, and carrying out their investigations by exploring the concepts, values, beliefs and assumptions embedded in their practice and in their description of it. Thus, as we can see from the chapters above, their intimate dramas which crystallise the dilemmas of their practice very quickly come to be seen as a core, and later, when they are apprehended in their wider context (both the wider context of the individual's professional incident and that wider context of the practice and traditions of their professions as a whole), they are seen as a small moral crisis and their significance recedes in the face of the greater weight of the wider professional problems uncovered in exploring it. Remarkably, too, when this process reveals itself as common across the chapters we see, just as we do in *Dubliners*, the human (and in this case professional) spirit struggling for survival in an alien climate. And although no writer actually articulates it like that, nevertheless the power of art to convey the ineffable or the un-nameable moves us to perceive that this is how it is for them.

Here, then, the research is not *using* autobiography as a tool to 'help with' or 'start off' the process in the form of incidents, anecdotes, diaries, journals (which is often how it is seen in humanistic enquiry). Rather, the autobiographical process – as known about in its literary genre including its struggles with objectivity, form shape, balance, style, image, reflection and introspection – *becomes* the research and enables the researcher to uncover a range of levels of analysis and interpretation of his or her practice and to attend with some justice to the complexity of personal–professional inter-relationships, decisions and judgements.

Here, too, the researcher–autobiographer becomes, like the artist, partly an outsider looking at his or her practice from afar, whilst being privy to the innermost thoughts about it too. It is no wonder that this provides an excellent basis for probing that most invisible capacity of all, which lies at the very heart of professionalism, namely professional judgement. In this sense what autobiographical research of this kind shows is professionals becoming more fully themselves. And it happens because they have put themselves and their practice in the centre of the frame and accepted the primacy of practice as the principle guiding all stages of their investigations. In the writing up of this it may mean presenting the critical incident at the point where it best allows its complexities to be understood irrespective of the chronology of the research action. It also means seeing the role of formal theory as a support in extending understanding of practice rather than as a directive in how to look at practice.

With these matters in mind, then, it is time to turn to the central detail of our response to Part Two.

References

Abbs, P. (1974). *Autobiography in Education*. Heinemann Educational.
Bottrall, M. (1958). *Every Man a Phoenix: Sudies in Seventeenth Century Autobiography*. John Murray.

Boud, D., Keogh, R. and Walker, D. (1985). *Reflection: Turning Experience into Learning*. Kogan Page.

Eisner, E. (1985). *The Art of Educational Evaluation*. Falmer Press.

Fish, D. *Appreciating Practice in the Caring Professions: Re-focusing Professional Development and Practitioner Research*. Butterworth–Heinemann. In press.

Ghiselin, B. (1956). The unity of *Dubliners*. In *James Joyce* Dubliners *and A Portrait of the Artist as a Young Man: a series of critical essays* (M. Beja, ed.), pp. 100–116. Macmillan.

Grumet, M. (1981). Restitution and reconstruction of educational experience: an autobiographical method for curriculum theory. In *Rethinking Curriculum Studies* (M. Lawn and L. Barton, eds.), pp. 115–130. Croom Helm.

Joyce, J. (1965 [1914]). *The Dubliners*. Jonathan Cape.

Pinar, W. (1986). 'Whole, bright, deep with understanding': issues in qualitative research and autobiographical method. In *Recent Developments in Curriculum Studies* (P. H. Taylor, ed.), pp. 6–24. NFER/Nelson.

Woods, P. (1987). Life histories and teacher knowledge. In *Educating Teachers: Changing the Nature of Pedagogical Knowledge* (J. Smyth, ed.), pp. 121–136. Falmer Press.

Chapter 12

A critical appreciation: attending to the voices of practitioners

The cases: overall intentions

In preparing each of the cases presented in the six chapters in Part Two the contributors worked as individual experts in their own practice to the common end of understanding that practice better and to noting within it the operation of professional judgement. Their cases are each cases of practitioners exploring their own professional practice which, for reasons set out in Part One, they see as characterised by artistry operating in a technical rational environment. Thus, each chapter is a journey in the development of one practitioner's understanding of individual practice viewed from within the wider context of professional artistry and understood in terms of the wider traditions of health care and a particular health care profession. As a result we have been made privy to individual insights, and, inevitably, we hear these through different voices. By attending to these voices we can appreciate more fully what is being said.

Apprehending the collection as a unity

To consider each study separately, however, is to overlook what they have to say, what can be learnt from them and the strengths they display, *as a unity*. The bases for claiming that they should be treated as a unity lies in the sense, which emerges across the writings, of shared format, shared context, shared aims and shared concerns. To see each chapter merely as an individual case is to ignore the ground swell of common elements, and the music of their combined voices, both of which add substantially to the weight of what is revealed.

The similarities between them are further reinforced by the fact that within their common remit they focus on slightly different subjects, interpret the demands of case study slightly differently and see with different eyes. This enables the sensitive reader to recognise how strongly their shared concerns come through despite the range of views, and to learn about the variety of emphasis which can emerge from different approaches to case study as a way of investigating personal professional practice. For example, within a general understanding of it, they view the significance of formal theory slightly differently and this influences their ability to link their individual case to the wider world of professional practice. Also, as we shall see in the following chapter, within a broad and shared understanding of the term 'professional judgement' they demonstrate divergent views about how it is operated. They thus offer as a collection, in ways that none could do alone, an overall exemplar of what can be achieved in insider practitioner research using the case study approach.

Appreciating the collection

This *collection* of individual chapters then is the focus and subject of our critical appreciation. We eschew the temptation to offer a reductionist analysis of this collection (categorising and quantifying components of the thinking it offers in an apparently objective way) and we wish to go beyond offering our interpretation (offering 'a view of' it by imposing our admittedly subjective meanings on it in order to explain it, find 'a message' in it or state what it has to say). We present instead what we believe is a thoughtful critical *response* to a collection of examples of professionals seeking better to understand their practices and their artistry. And we do so by seeking to understand the collection by any and as many means as possible (while accepting that there may always be more means to understanding it than have been operated and as many ways to appreciate it as there are human beings to do the appreciating), and attempting, so far as our inevitably subjective reading allows, to let its content and artistry speak for itself.

In so doing we are consciously providing an example of the appreciation of practice and of a study of practice. That is, we are seeking to illustrate an additional way in which practitioners might in future attend to the artistry in their *own* practice and their own presentation of it, or of how they might explore the work of colleagues in a critical friendship.

We have already, in Part One and in Chapter 11, sought to set this collection in a context that helps us to make sense of it. We shall now attempt to open up the writing before you, the reader, and enable you to see in this collection of professional stories the significance below the surface and to discern the whispers of what lies just beyond its voiced details. In order to do so we have already, of course, scrutinised each chapter in very considerable detail, seeking to understand what each writer is offering, seeking its themes and insights, looking at its elements, noting its form and structure as well as its focus and setting and its style and imagery. And in so doing we recognise and acknowledge our own subjectivities, values, assumptions, beliefs, interests – and the fact that we have of course also played another role in all this, as editors of this book. That is, we have had the final control over the org-anisation of this collection within the larger context of this book, and it is to this that we turn first.

The organisation of the collection

The organisation of the chapters in this collection as presented in Part Two was decided only after they had all been written. In making our decisions about this final order we were far less concerned about highlighting the fact that these are views from different professions than about how the chapters exemplified the themes of this book. In that sense we attempted to do what our contributors also aim at – to look at alternative perspectives on our focus of interest (as indicated in Part One) and also to keep faith with our own vision, which is about arguing for a different kind of practitioner research and professional education than is currently common in heath care, and arguing for the particular importance of professional judgement in understanding and developing profes-sional practice.

Our rationale for the sequence of these chapters is, then, as follows. We offer first a chapter which in itself previews the themes and processes to come. We follow this with a number of contrasting chapters which offer some but not all elements of the kind of reflective autobiographical research, professional development and insight into professional judgement that we are trying to illustrate. We place at the end of the collection a chapter which takes a slightly more distanced and therefore a 'longer' view of the issues and processes we are interested in. By chance this order also provides us with a series of views from contrasting health care professions, and we believe that this is also a strength of the collection.

In choosing this order we have produced an overall shape to the collection which is in a sense organic rather than linear. That is, we have offered a whole whose shape grows from within rather than something which has a hierarchical order or contains a simple chronological set of relationships between elements. The structure of the collection then is appropriate, we would argue, to its overall content – as a whole view of professional practice – and to the variety of perspectives that need to be considered in case study. And in this respect we have also paralleled the structure of the individual chapters which grew organically, with the particular role of the critical incident being placed wherever it best enabled writers to display the understandings gained. Indeed, we believe that an organic structure as seen both within and across the collection is almost inevitable given the complexity and messiness of professional practice.

In detail, in terms of order this means that Rosemary's chapter is placed first because in her work we find the themes and processes to come and we believe that it provides readers with a clear overview of what we mean by autobiographical (or insider practitioner) research using a case study approach. It highlights tensions between bureaucratic and humanistic issues, between formal theory, personal theory and practice, between artistry and rationalism, between personal and professional responses to situations, between scientific and interpretative enquiry, and between good and poor professional judgements, in health care. It also demonstrates the processes and their importance of theorising practice, of crystal-lising professional insights, of thinking critically about practice and of capturing all this in case study. Rosemary's chapter achieves all this by offering a professional incident in nursing from the point of view of the consumer, and rapidly turns this into the means of reflecting on and learning about professional practice including her own. Professional judgement lies at the heart of many of the decisions here presented, and she shows how her understanding in respect of this is developed.

Crissi's chapter follows. It provides an example – this time from occupational therapy – of how the vitally important affective elements of professional life (which in this case are a response to the almost unbearable tensions endemic to professional practice) can render practice complex or even get in the way of professional judgement.

Richard's work (of a consultant in palliative care) is focused exclusively in the arena of professional practice and offers us some uncomfortable reflections on judgements which he made during his work. These he seeks to interpret without the benefit of formal theory in this field, leaving the reader to provide some of these perspectives (which perhaps earlier sections of this book might in part have equipped readers to be able to do).

We have placed Sheila's chapter to provide a contrast to Richard's and roughly at the heart of the collection because she offers some fascinating parallels between the problems she has in her own research in this chapter and those of the nurse practitioner student she is supporting who is conducting orthodox undergraduate research. We thus see her portraying many of the issues which we raise in the early parts of this book.

Judith's chapter shares with us the painful voyage of a physiotherapist turned educator seeking technical rational answers to the essentially problematic dilemmas of assessment – particularly she highlights the tensions central to trying to develop assessment processes which are fair, educational and useful bureaucratically. We see her finally coming to recognise that she must seek a balance between these and live with the nature of uncertainty which is endemic to professional artistry in both education and professional practice.

Clive's writing oscillates between his own teaching (working in staff development mode with a group of professionals) and his own return to professional practice in nursing in order to explore judgements about a particularly intimate and difficult professional matter. The distancing that comes from a sense that he belongs totally in neither arena allows him to consider judgement in slightly more objective terms. But his work also shows the need for far more understanding to be developed about professional judgement, and as such acts both as an end and a beginning.

The shape of the collection, then, with its outer two slightly broader studies binding together those within, shows, through their differences, something of the shared perceptions of the contributors. But there is further unity too. All contributors were working at one shared problem about how best to approach the investigation of their own practice – what traditions of enquiry they were working in and how to attend to matters like validity and what counted as rigour – and with one main shared problem about processes – how to make sense of their practice. The following two sections elaborate upon these.

Investigating practice: case study

We have offered arguments for the case study approach that we encouraged colleagues to adopt, and the details of what this tradition of investigation entails, in Chapter 3 (and further details again can be found in Fish, in press). From what we have offered above it will have become clear that case study is itself an art (see also Stake, 1995). As such it was something which our contributors found very different from the ideas about 'proper research' that many of them brought with them (even when they were well aware of survey, illuminative and action research). In fact writing a case study was something that they learnt to do as they went along, and certainly the community spirit which quickly sprang up amongst them supported them in this. They fairly quickly came to recognise that case study does not follow rigid routines, that they needed to find their own ways into it and through it, and that beyond the guidelines we offered them it was something that they needed to grapple with and interpret for themselves. There are a number of places at which they overtly recognise this in their writing.

The one other set of issues that caused many of them concern, working as they do in arenas where research traditions are still almost entirely rooted in the positivistic paradigm, were about the validity, reliability and rigour of their work and how this could be provided for within case study. Again, Golby helps us here, pointing out that what needs to be guarded against are matters where bias can creep in, atypical events are taken as typical, and there are false inferences and shaky generalisations (see Golby, 1993). These

matters are safeguarded where the possibility of bias is acknowledged, the matters of generalisation are handled as already
discussed, arguments are laid out clearly, sources of evidence and
what they are taken as evidence of are clearly cited and values and
assumptions are uncovered. Some of this is taken care of within the
theorising of practice as we have conceived it, and some is a matter
of normal scholarly rigour as found in any proper academic study.
Openness is essential, as is the provision of enough detail for the
reader to reconstruct the issues and reconsider the conclusions.
Only the reader can judge these finally. And it is the reader too who
can attest to the consistency of argument, findings, and tone and
recognise their authenticity, deeming the work reliable by the
number of chords it seems to strike with their own experience. All
writers sought too, to validate their own work by offering careful
and explicit documentation of their work, by recognising the
perspectives of others involved in their practice, and by quoting
views from formal theory.

For this reason, the contributors came to agree that the rigour of
work of this kind is discovered by the writers and found by the
readers as being *in the writing*. It is *in* the process of writing that
they learnt about the artistry of their work, learnt to describe and
to theorise their practice – in short learnt the disciplines of collecting
their thoughts, ordering their understanding and presenting their
case with artistry. And it is in response to the quality of the writing,
too, that readers recognise the reverberations of life as they too
know it, and find a sense of wholeness – of 'completeness' as Golby
calls it (Golby, 1993, p. 29).

Contributors, then, experienced a growing understanding about
case study as they worked on their drafts over a period of many
months. But they also shared one other common worry. Having
crystallised their practical problem in a first draft of their critical
incident, and recognised that their practice contains much more
that is professional artistry than is technical rational, contributors
quickly came up against the problem about how to make sense of
this complexity that was their practice.

Theorising practice: a common approach and processes

We argued (as we have said in Chapter 3) that 'it is by being
theorised that practice gains its meaning'. We offered all our contri-

butors particular support in this area and certainly believe that their case studies show that they came to focus more sharply than most had done before on theorising their practice. We shared with them the idea that this means 'an active uncovering of the thoughts, assumptions, beliefs and values that lie beneath practice'. And we show below many examples of this – where they reveal in a controlled and balanced way the depth of thought and feeling lying beneath at least some of their actions. They can also be seen as recognising honestly the *results* within their practice of their assumptions, reasoning, values, beliefs, judgements and actions. They certainly identify some of the problematic and contestable issues and some of the dilemmas endemic in their practice. Of course the further one goes in this direction the more painful it can become, and there is clear evidence in their work that it became painful, but there is also clear evidence that they gained a great deal in understanding their practice and themselves better as a result of this. Their recognition of the wellsprings of their judgements, decisions, reasoning and actions are therefore the subject of our appreciation.

If these then are the common characteristics of the collection at a general level, we now need to attend to our appreciation of the work in more detail.

In terms of that important characteristic of art, the close relationship of content and form, we have already demonstrated that the overall collection has a shape which is appropriate to the overall content. We shall now attempt to do justice to the individual cases and their relationship within the collection, and to illustrate that each chapter too has its own form and structure which relate appropriately to the content being offered.

The parts and the whole: content, form and structure

In terms of both form and content, one striking characteristic shared by each case study is that all writers come to the conclusion that there is no conclusion. This is an inevitable insight of writing autobiography where the ending must, by definition, be unfinished. Lack of an obvious ending is also found typically in many art forms in the twentieth century.

Examples of this include Richard's comment that there are no solutions to his problems, except to formulate new theories for going forward. Rosemary says her thinking will go on, she resolves to keep person-centred, humanistic and holistically oriented values as a central focus for students and in her practice as a teacher. Crissi shows how important it is for professional development to be able to unravel and to face the complexities of personally uncomfortable situations of the kind professionals prefer to push under the carpet. And we have a strong sense that she will continue to show this courage when difficulties occur. Clive shows that the use of professional judgement is complex and that the challenge facing us all is to make expert practice explicit and show that it cannot be standardised. Sheila's final sub-heading indicates that her conclusions are not the end, declares that the process of reflection and attempting to understand and refine practice will never end, and that she will continue to learn from her single incident. Judith resolves to face up to the uncertainty and the inevitable tensions in assessment and to work to develop assessment schemes that are more flexible and which will be responsive to evolving changes in education. In Judith's words, all recognise that 'the understandings and insights gained will influence deeply their future practice'.

Beyond this, the detail of the chapters shows how the contributors have each shaped their work so that there is indeed a unity between form and content. The form in three of these chapters, whilst still being relatively straightforward, has nevertheless been developed well beyond the linear presentation of a simple story simply narrated. The other three offer examples of greater complexity of form, each of which neatly reinforces the ebb and flow of the reflections being presented.

Rosemary provides us with her incident at the beginning of her work, and although she is surprised by the results of some of her explorations, and comes upon some insights unexpectedly, she is clearly in control of the various themes which emerge from her incident and this enables the reader to grasp them easily. The essential simplicity of her structure (which begins with her incident and circles round it exploring it in ever widening ripples) is a necessary vehicle for the complexity and interrelationship of the ideas she is grappling with in what is a highly interpretative case study which uses critical reflection and raises matters for deliberation. Crissi also weaves a circle round her incident, coming back to it again and again, initially showing the difficulty she has with finding her way through the affective maze which comes between her and her practice, and gradually establishing new understandings of her personal dilemmas through further and later reflections. Richard tells his story simply, recording his comments as he goes, and taking up the whole chapter with narrative. His is a story which demonstrates his own theorising in rather more chronological terms. But he prepares the reader very carefully for this at the beginning by spending time setting the very important context.

By contrast to these examples of relatively simple relationships between form and content, Sheila offers us throughout her chapter an almost rhythmic approach to and retreat from the anger her incident generated in her. This rhythm is at first almost imperceptible, but grows in visibility as the chapter proceeds. Further, and parallel to this structure, we are permitted to see in Sheila's thinking an early movement towards and retreat from the recognition that she and her student are doing similar and yet different things. All her students are required to undertake a practice-based research project to provide an assessment for the course. The student who seeks Sheila's help is carrying out action research to 'develop and improve an aspect of her clinical practice' but is not having much success in writing it up because she recognised that she did not understand the processes she had used. A little later Sheila says of herself: 'I recently decided to confront one of the incidents [of my practice] in order to understand it better and to ... improve my professional activity and behaviour.' Thus the student is seeking to change her practice through a politically oriented research form in which we suspect she is looking for answers about how to do it better. She is also looking, as Sheila says, a little later, to get a pass – to do work acceptable to the examiners and (at the bottom of the list) to learn something of use in her practice.

In contrast to her student, Sheila is first and foremost seeking to understand her practice by reflecting on a detailed incident from it, with a belief that as a result of understanding it better she will improve her professional work. She is 'not necessarily searching for a solution but rather trying to understand'. She is also producing a chapter in a book which will itself not entirely please her 'examiners' – that is, her own university research administration and the next university research assessment exercise, which on past form, will be looking for more positivistic work. So she has chosen to enlighten her understanding at some cost. There are some fascinating parallels here between student's and tutor's research work, but also striking divergences in their approaches to research. And all this the reader is permitted to see before the writer herself becomes aware of it.

But there is more. The student's problem generates worries in Sheila about the different agendas for the student research module of which she has charge. She recognises her own uncertainty about the purpose of the research dissertation, the conflict between learning about research and the course's 'assessment agenda', and, most irking of all perhaps, the sense that to change the module's focus would require considerable changes in the perception of colleagues and examiners. She then comes with what is almost a shout of surprise upon a number of insights. She comes to a realisation about the primacy of practice as a result of reading an article by Landgrebe and Winter, and decides to look afresh at her practical incident. Having cleared away all the issues that have clouded her thinking, she is then struck by the parallels which she uncovers and which the reader has already been allowed to deduce. She then concludes, 'I have gained insights which have undoubtedly developed me personally as well as professionally.' Amongst these are a recognition of the need to accept and work with the problems of practice and be less stressed by its uncertainties. These insights have come because she learnt *during* the writing of this chapter to abandon her attempt to analyse her incident in favour of reflecting upon it, and secondly because she turns back from formal theory to look more closely at practice.

Interestingly, Judith has her own structure for setting out and exploring her critical incident (which she places at the end of her chapter). But she also recognises that readers may need to be free to come at her material in a simpler way, and so invites them if they feel the need to seek out and read first the incident that crystallised her dilemmas. She, too, adds additional sections to her story as it unfolds to enrich it with later reflections. This is partly because she takes a rather more didactic approach to the reader, presenting her work as a means of helping readers. She also shows us that her original expectations (influenced by a technical rational approach to research), were that the structure of her chapter would be linear and simple (that it would proceed by means of presenting the event, reflecting upon it, generating questions, following these through with theoretical explorations and concluding with how the exercise has altered her practice). Here she recognises the struggle she had to come to terms with the nature of professional artistry and the need to take a holistic approach to the research and its presentation. Quoting Postel, she draws attention quite early in her chapter to the need to attend to the whole of experience and to recognise the influence of past experiences on current behaviour, but she only makes this notion her own towards the end of her writing. Thus, the structure of her chapter is truly organic.

Judith's chapter also moves with the rhythm of her progress in understanding the problems at the heart of assessment. About half way through she comes to a core insight about assessment being essentially an administrative and political tool rather than an educational one and about trying to mark scholarly work with a clinical hat on, but then backs away from articulating this, taking her thinking round again to the puzzles involved and ending with an awareness that she still has not resolved all the tensions but is learning to live with them. (Perhaps it is rather that, as she half guesses but never quite says, assessment is rather more concerned with administrative and political purposes and is rather less interested in being utterly fair, equitable or educational, the former being easier to achieve in a technical rational climate.) She also calls attention to an interesting parallel between the development of understanding about assessment in her *profession* at profession-wide level and the development of her *own* individual under-standing of it.

Clive reports on his work with practising professionals and his return to professional practice to investigate a particularly sensitive aspect of professionalism. As a result he has some interesting points to raise about judgement. We shall take these up in detail in the final chapter of this section. For now it is interesting to note that Clive is the only writer who adopts a model for helping his reflections on his own practice and which he uses to shape his writing. Interestingly, in the event, it seems to be more of a hindrance than a help. He also shares his initial awkwardness in returning to practice and reports that thinking about practice got in the way of doing. In both cases what he comes to discover is the importance of attending to practice itself and not some chimera of it. The structure of his chapter leads us finally to this revelation.

There are many issues in all chapters relating to professional judgement and the final chapter of this critical appreciation will discuss these in detail.

Focus and setting

The comparisons and contrasts in focus and setting wrought by placing these chapters as we have, perhaps also enable us to view them as contrasting portraits in a whole collection rather than simply a series of otherwise unrelated entities.

Thus we can see that in Rosemary's work the focal point is the broad perspective of a practitioner seeing professional dilemmas holistically as a result of reflecting on one incident. The lens then adjusts to a series of narrower examples of practitioners concentrating on the affective, the practical and the research dimension, before moving back out to a longer-distance consideration of unresolvable dilemmas central to the education of practitioners, and coming ultimately to an overview of the complexities of practitioners' judgement.

There are common focuses here in terms of the dilemmas of practice which demand a response. What is expected of all health care practitioners is expert *action* – immediate action – underpinned, of course, by expert knowledge. Health care practitioners are always being pressed into action and their training seeks to equip them for it, when in fact what you are is probably more important than (and equips you better for) what you do. All the writers show in their different ways how they feel this unbearable burden of expectation and how seeking understanding of a piece of practice enables them to come to accept it, see it in perspective, and see beyond it. And beyond and behind all this there is an overall focus across all the chapters on professional judgement. As we shall see in the next and final chapter of this section, each contributor's chapter is a journey in the development of understanding about professional judgement – even when they are not exactly articulated as such.

In this sense, then, the critical incidents themselves, which have prompted these deeper understandings, are less significant than perhaps their writers originally felt and thought. They have perhaps been put back into perspective via the very processes of enquiry the writers went through and so by the time we see them in their final place in each chapter they have receded into the overall picture.

To be sure, we see behind Rosemary's controlled words 'dismay, disbelief and consternation' and 'almost disbelief' a horror and disgust in relation to how her parents were treated in hospital. And we see in her own subsequent reactions of not complaining and of being tempted to weave her story into her educational offering to nurse students, the conflict between the ideal and the real, theory and practice, personal theory and formal theory, personal reaction and professional response. And it is true that these conflicts are echoed in the critical incidents of each subsequent chapter. We see Crissi's disbelief and distress about how her first year practitioners were behaving and about what she was hearing in the subsequent management meeting, but it is how she makes meaning of all this that is of real interest. We are aware of Richard's discomfort about his actions, feelings and judgements in several incidents related to a dying patient, but it is how he sees his practice more generally that we seek to hear. We are privy to Sheila's amazement at her anger when caught up in the middle of professional commitments by the need to attend immediately to a student in difficulties, but it is the issues that this raises about research that are of central interest. We see the deeper dilemmas of assessment in Judith's alarm when a student appealed against her mark, and in her repeated disappointments at failing to crack assessment. Behind Clive's descriptions of practice we are aware of his partially acknowledged discomfort at the way theory and theorising got in the way of his understanding nursing practice and in the way of his writing it up! Thus it is not the incidents themselves that matter so much as the serious, disciplined enquiry into them that has uncovered the insights and understandings for the writers and for us. For this reason the incidents *themselves* did not figure in our rationale for ordering the chapters in this collection.

Our judgement as editors about order was, however, also affected by the fact that the settings in the chapters range widely across professions and that this is useful from the point of view of gaining a more general view of issues in health care. They begin with a comparison of hospital and community nursing and health visiting and their implications for the education of nurses. They move through issues in post-registration support and management in occupational therapy. The setting then changes to work in the hospital, the consultant's hospice and the home in support of a dying patient. In a new twist the setting becomes the research arena itself with a nurse education slant. We then turn to a view behind the scenes in physiotherapy education. Finally we find ourselves in a split setting between the classroom and 'real' practice in nursing.

Overall themes: major motifs

We have argued then that the work of the contributors in Part Two constitutes more than a portfolio of autobiographical sketches and also more than a series of small scale case studies of professional practice. It is, rather, an overall composition which presents as a unity some reflective and deliberative writings of practitioners in a range of health care professions from the final decade of the twentieth century. In other words, by virtue of the timing of its publication and as a result of its content, it can be seen as a *fin de siècle* doxography (a compilation of deep thoughts, feelings and opinions) which gives the reader some sense of the state of the health care professions at this time as viewed by some practitioners who, of course, by their very contribution to this work can be said to embrace particular and shared values but who are also senior and experienced members of their professions. And these case studies gain their ultimate validity as they cause deep reverberations in the reader who has also 'been there'.

This sense of the reader both recognising and being privy to deep thinking and acute sensitivities comes out of the fact that these reflections on personal practice are written in autobiographical form. Here reflective practice is demonstrated as an art in its own right. Richard finds it uncomfortable (which of course all learning is) and refers to it as 'an attitude of mind which once embraced can never be abandoned', and as a journey involving 'hard and emotional work, exhausting but exciting'. Crissi makes her excruciating personal feelings tangible and the reader experiences them alongside her as the chapter progresses. Rosemary provides us with a calm professional exterior through which we are allowed to discern her strong reactions and a turmoil of thoughts which seem the more powerful for being held in check. Judith hopes to illustrate the processes of her reflection so that readers can draw on them for their own use, by singling out, in special sections, insights that occurred during reflection. Clive too is seeking to encourage others to explore the deeper meanings of their own practice and to raise questions about a whole range of issues, as he himself does. He argues that we should take time to contemplate the deeper meanings of our practices and to uncover what they can tell us. He contrasts this with both standing back from practice in a distanced, objective, technical rational way which will not help us to improve practice, and with working on the basis of intuition, which unless it is explored will never become insight.

This overall scope and focus of the compilation is reinforced by three major and interrelated motifs, or dominant themes, to which each chapter contributes but which only the whole collection presents fully. It captures some experiences and difficulties of practitioners as they work in and investigate their practice and crystallises something of the flavour of the moral and spiritual condition of professional practice in health care in the 1990s, which is perhaps the primary theme of this collection. It also illustrates the agonising which is endemic to the exercising by practitioners of both professional judgement and responsible action (as we shall see in the final section of this chapter). At the same time it underlines the desperate need in pre-registration and post-registration courses for the next millennium to nourish, support and educate professional judgement and its consequence – morally defensible action. We shall now attempt to point up some recurring themes which underscore and elaborate upon these major motifs.

Themes and sub-themes

The primary theme then – that of the moral and spiritual state of professional practice in health care and of the experience of working as a reflective practitioner within it – finds its expression in the frequent (but un-pre-planned) repetition across chapters (and therefore also found across professions) of some sub-themes which illustrate the current tensions and antitheses which practitioners have to live with or try to appear to reconcile in their work. These tensions particularly revolve around the technical rational versus the professional artistry view of professionalism and all the conflicting values that this issue brings with it. They also include the demands made by unresolvable moral and human dilemmas and the diminishing grip on the human side of professionalism in the face of the technological revolution. Along with these go the fast pace of change and the frustrations of the impossibility of being able to communicate with the public when professional complexities are expected to be comprehended from the brief 'sound bites' which are all that are offered to health professionals by the media.

These recurrent themes give colour and atmosphere to the collection, indicating a deep sense of unease, of distress and of moral dilemma amongst practitioners which seems to be leading the professions almost to a state of torpor. Much of this seems to have grown out of the conflict between practitioners' professional views and concerns and the public expectations which have been shaped by the materialism and consumerism of the last decades of the twentieth century.

All writers are to a greater or lesser extent overtly aware of the political, social and moral context of their practice. Rosemary calls attention to the major significance of context for understanding practice and its influence on professional practice, emphasising that meanings are socially constructed and that the meanings we give to experience are not fixed but vary according to the circumstances and the time of our reflection. She is acutely aware of the values and beliefs at work in the personal and social context of her story. Sheila refers to the broader social and cultural context of her own and her students' practice, questions the social and professional functions of a school of nursing and is on the brink of probing the moral issues in her own labelling of her student as poor and lazy. Crissi refers to today's bureaucratic approach within the NHS, and shows us how the almost ritualistic workings of a particular committee can result not just in insensitivities but in missing the point altogether. Judith becomes aware of the administrative and political dimensions of assessment, notes the changes in the meaning of assessment across different cultures and across the years, and shows how the history of her profession's attitude to assessment is parallel to her own. Richard's awareness of the importance of context in understanding his story is shown in the care he takes to set the scene at the start of his chapter and in his comments about pragmatism and the political climate and the ethics of his actions and their moral consequences for the GP and future patients. He also notes that his critical incident is just one variant in a long line of uncommon but important incidents. Clive becomes concerned about ethical and moral considerations in his responsibility for patients and in his profession as a whole.

Endemic to the overall themes and motifs then, are deep conflicts in respect of values, beliefs and assumptions. All writers are aware of and draw attention to their assumptions, and many, like Judith, admit that theirs were mostly unexamined until they reflected on their actions. She uncovers the assumptions she had been making about the objectivity of assessment based on her own earlier experience, and exposes her false belief that the problems emanating from assessment were really the students' lack of understanding. Sheila of course has a similar problem with her student. She also probes the notion of care and the values that lie behind it, noting that it differs in an educational environment from a clinical one, and notes that professional behaviour is partly determined by life history and experience. Crissi demonstrates the differences in values between herself and her newly qualified 'participants', and is herself surprised by how powerful are the values inculcated in the pre-registration course. Richard tries to cut through his own assumptions about how others might see him, as does Sheila. Sheila also notes that there are often both personal and institutional conflicts of value in relationship to adult learning, and recognises with distaste how much the curriculum she operates is assessment led with no apparent room for students' critical thinking.

Rosemary has much to say about conflicting and competing values. She points out as she talks of community-related values that sometimes it is necessary to recognise sympathetically that different values operate in different settings because of the complexity of particular circumstances. She also makes the point that 'the way we would *like* to practise is not the same as the way we *do*', and she notes that values can be compromised in the battle to retain a job and that her own values are not easily achievable in institutional settings. (Sheila too says 'I could no longer ignore the gulf between what I believe about practice and what I do in reality ... which made me see my practice in a new light.') Rosemary also draws attention to the way values are influenced by experiences, and notes that they are politically influenced and that no knowledge is value-free. She agonises over professional responsibilities in respect of all this in a very moving passage on pages 80–90 and makes the powerful point that the risk in terms of values would seem to be in their denial rather than in their recognition.

The most common sub-theme is probably about the pressures from the public and from government for objectivity (resultant from the climate in which positivism is the only god of our age, whose assumptions have become endemic to and unchallenged in all our thinking). And related to this is the frustration of knowing or learning of the inevitability of subjectivity in the reality of professional practice. This tension of course is always endemic to professional practice but is currently emphasised by the value systems imposed upon professionals in the last decade of the twentieth century. They currently seem designed to leave the professional with an unenviable choice of whether to collude with the public view or to feel guilty about not accepting it, but as we suggested in Chapter 1, it results in professionals feeling under siege.

In every chapter of this collection, then, we see the tension between the objectivity required by public, governments and even by professionalism itself, and the subjectivity which is all that in reality practitioners can experience and which emerges in their writing as a result of the personal nature of the investigations and the autobiographical form in which they are reported. It is also interesting that some writers had been brought up to consider it inappropriate to use the first person singular in academic writing and that they are not entirely comfortable with it. Thus, Judith, whose relationship with the reader is slightly self-conscious as a result of being unfamiliar with writing in the first person, talks of being driven to make assessment as objective as possible, and of 'flawless objectivity', and shows how she believed that any part of clinical performance could be clearly defined and measured objectively. She shows us her struggles in accommodating ideas about the subjectivity of assessment. Rosemary faces squarely the importance of the personal and the subjective, and yet her felt need to articulate this says much about how little accepted it still is in her world. By contrast Richard quietly asserts his right against those who would refuse to recognise that there are elements of the personal in our professional judgements, and Clive also feels the need to warn the reader against interpreting in the current fashion the processes of his investigation of his practice as 'objective or disembodied'.

Related to this sub-theme are two additional sets of tensions – the tensions between the personal and affective response to a situation and the professional ideal of detached and calm behaviour, and also the distinctions between working as an individual and as a member of a community. Crissi tries hard to stay calm in the face of provocation during her critical incident and during the subsequent 'critical' meeting, and only brings her complaining participants up short when she abandons this approach (when her patience finally snaps) in favour of getting them to see her point of view for a change. Sheila too feels she has failed by becoming angry. But Rosemary points out that not far below the surface of supposedly professional incidents is a person trying to make sense of and understand what occurred. And indeed, all contributors seem amongst other things to offer extended illustrations of this very point. It is also she who, bringing her interesting community background to her nursing practice and her scholarly work, sought in her masters degree and in her reference to formal theory in her chapter, to belong to a community of like-minded thinkers, and who also reacts against the closed community of the hospital. But there are issues about community lying behind each chapter even where they are not made explicit. And all this illustrates Rosemary's sense of the taken for granted which, when given closer attention, reveals itself as problematic.

Beyond these sub-themes the following seem to highlight themselves by their frequency:

- the confusion as to where practitioners' understanding about practice comes from
- the mistaken expectation that practitioners are all-knowing and utterly certain experts
- the contrasts between action and various kinds of theory, between action and inaction or exhaustion, frustration or dull routine
- the contrast between the theory of what practitioners are taught and the reality of health care practice
- the contrast between the controls imposed upon practitioners and the freedom necessary to exercise professional action and judgement
- the distinction between the taken for granted and the problematic
- the acute awareness in all of this of the importance of looking at professional work as a whole as against the requirements to consider it a series of discrete units or skills

- the difference in professional practice between appearance and reality, fraud and probity, unawareness and insight, illumination and confusion.

It is interesting to note that this list starts with and ends with the word 'confusion'.

An example of how even apparent insight can prove treacherous is shown when Sheila comes to a partial insight about how to help her student (by sending her some literature) and when Judith comes to what she later realises was a mistaken belief about assessment. Judith and Crissi are each unhappy about being a fraud – 'appearing as an expert yet having no explicit or sound basis for my judgement'. Judith also recognises that she might have been encouraging students to develop superficial learning habits and that the very guidelines for assessment could have a negative affect on their learning. But it is Rosemary who voices the issues about the role of interpretation in these matters, neatly reminding us that our understandings or meanings are all a process of interpretation and that professional knowledge itself can be used (or misused) as a means of domination, or be a tool to produce inappropriate dependence or ill-founded faith.

In addition to all this there is the ubiquitous problem of communication which results, as Rosemary points out, from listener and speaker working on different agendas and listening but not hearing, or as Sheila points out 'communicating one message verbally and the opposite in my actions'. This contrasts with the ideal of showing respect for patients and clients and operating in communicative partnership with them and their families. Crissi's chapter illustrates the problems of communication between herself and the unresponsive participants in her programme. In all this, writers are grappling with the visible and invisible parts of professional practice, and it is Clive who points this up in his memorable image of the iceberg: 'Expert clinical practice is like an iceberg, with one tenth on show.' It is getting at the nine tenths which is invisible – ineffable – that is attended to by treating practice as an art. (This is a crucial point which we shall return to in the concluding section of this book.)

Similarly, there emerges from the chapters a chorus of anxiety about the burden of the demand for practitioners to be know-ledgeable experts in contrast to the reality of their extensive uncertainties. The nature and basis of this knowledge and expertise clearly needs to be more carefully thought through, but there is no doubt that the pressure is felt as almost intolerable in the face of many unknowns in practice. And ironically one uncertainty is where the improved understanding of practice itself can come from. Many of the writers take time to recognise that it comes in the main from looking more deeply at their practice. Thus they have to fight their way away from the temptation to find and quote 'the right' formal theory, and to cope with the naked feelings resulting from not rushing off at the start to conduct a literature search. They have rather to recognise that it is necessary to wait until they have unearthed their real questions (after which a literature search is more appropriate) and also to see that theory needs to play a quite different role in their thinking and writing. Sheila's discomfort is palpable as she recognises her uncertainty about the very purpose of the undergraduate research dissertation, the support of which lies at the very heart of one of her major professional responsibilities. She is led too, to question her beliefs about teaching and learning and neatly turns Carper's well-known text for nursing, which lists four ways of knowing, into ways of unknowing.

Importantly, gradually in each of the chapters and therefore in the collection as a whole, these unknowns begin to be recognised as far more positive and valuable than the previous unfounded assumptions. But there is a sense that there is far more work to be done before this is more generally accepted in the professions themselves.

There is a confusion, too, about where professional knowledge comes from. Crissi shows how what had been communicated to her 'participants' during their pre-registration course actually got in the way of (and perhaps made more difficult) their hearing or making new meanings during practice. Sheila offers to send the student some articles which were relevant to the undergraduate's problem, but later discovers during her own enquiries that learning to understand practice comes from looking at practice (thus discovering the meaning behind the already known words about the primacy of practice). Richard and Rosemary also note the importance and uniqueness of practice, and Rosemary indicates importantly that solving practical problems does not always lead to increased understanding, while Clive has clearly been influenced (in our view misguidedly) by those published nursing standards that regard understanding as a *skill*. There is a sense behind these discoveries that, as Sheila articulates, they are taking her out of kilter with the orthodoxies of her profession. And Richard notes that those who adopt the role of expert and subscribe to professional rivalries may be prevented from entering into co-operative partnerships with colleagues.

The inevitable conclusion from all this is that balancing these imperatives is the delicate work of all professionals but that this can only be achieved with confidence where the inherent contradictions of the work of a professional have been recognised and, along with self-knowledge, accepted as part of the richness of professional life.

Certainly their reflections on their critical incidents raise in contributors' minds questions about theory (personal and formal, espoused and theory-in-use) and issues about research of this kind (which involves working towards new understanding). For example, we see all the writers struggling out of the bondage of technical rational and positivist thinking. We also see how this makes them less comfortable with the technical rational world of professional practice that they all inhabit. Judith, for example, shows how she was trapped in the endless attempt to tighten the guidelines for marking because they did not work, and how she needed to know that each marker was marking consistently and admits (with a sense of exhaustion) even three quarters of the way through her writing that she may need to develop yet more levels of competencies for assessment. She shows how she took time to break out of these vicious circles, and suggests that in the end it is the exhaustion itself, and the recognition that competencies fail to capture the more abstract elements and professional qualities she values, that makes her do so – but that even then she has to live in a world where quality controls exert pressure to regularise marking. Judith concludes that the process of reflection has influenced the way she will assess in future more than any formal theory ever has. Sheila too opens up similar problems and refers to her personal theories. Clive fights against the positivistic, notes that the measurable evidence of practice is small, and suggests that the world of 'objective evidence, outcome measures and random controlled trials simply shrugs its shoulders at the messy, unquantifiable nature of professional artistry'. But, of course, ignoring it does not mean that it will go away.

One bastion of authority that all contributors to Part Two have now to come to terms with is, of course, formal theory. How they use it is therefore interesting. Judith and Crissi, for example, use it to validate, confirm and enlighten their ideas. Crissi shows her changing ideas about formal theory and when and where to turn to it, contrasting her approach in this chapter to that in her masters dissertation. Judith boldly reports early in her chapter that her conclusions support the work of one theorist. But she also satirises herself in this respect as one who, seeking answers leapt frantically from one formal theory to another, whilst ignoring her own personal theory. She quickly comes to the idea that formal theory is not easily or simply put into practice, but even at the end she is excited to find a new theory which accounts for some of her problems with assessment. Richard writes freely without the benefit of theory (but perhaps as a result seems to take his reflections less far), Clive bases his work on a model, which in the end gets in his way. He also voices his dilemma about whether to have looked at the literature before entering the practice. He says that in a research study the design itself would help to clarify this. In fact he does choose to turn to the literature first and to consider his own practice beside the theory. He adds in a short but piquant sentence: 'In fact the literature helped very little', and reflects how many times existing literature does not 'fit' practice. Sheila too discovers that she needs to look at her practice first (because in practice there are no absolute truths or certainties). Rosemary on the other hand uses formal theory for a range of purposes associated with helping her to think critically, and explicitly rejects models as reductionist. She is most explicit about the role of formal theory in her practice and her reflections on practice. She aims at reflective *critical* enquiry and seems uncomfortable about starting writing without carrying out a literature survey (and such an omission is of course unorthodox), but she shows a great facility for bringing to mind relevant literature even during her practice. (A literature survey, as she said when she saw these comments, should be triggered by the questions raised in the case as a result of reflection upon practice, rather than pre-empting it.) She calls attention to the theory–practice gap between *A Vision of the Future* and nursing practice, and (very properly in our view) makes the point firmly that making links with formal theory has shed further light on her practice. She enjoys being part of a community of thinking, and theory enables her to see her work in this way.

There is much in this writing too about control versus freedom. The sense of constraint and control, because practitioners' actions have been prescribed, is in stark contrast with the need for freedom of choice and principle if decision-making is to be professional as opposed to technical. This is felt deeply by all the writers, as is their need to combat the untidiness of practice. Sheila describes herself as the sort of person who likes neatness and being in control, and, although she knows that practice is messy, she feels she has failed if hers is so. She demonstrates the ability to hold incompatible views when she says that she believes that her own success or failure lies under her own control, but that in reality many things are outside that control, and when she balances the autonomy of the learner against the control of the teacher. Similarly, in Rosemary's writing there is, as she herself points out, much about control versus independence, and about ring fences, imprisonment, bondage and escape. Crissi too talks of control, of the participants, of her frustrations, and of taking back control of the programme. She also vividly describes how she feels 'imprisoned' with the complaining participants, about being 'trapped', about her colleagues' 'congratulating her on her escape' from the NHS. In Richard's writing too there is a sense of release in being able to talk about his practice in a reflective mode, and from Judith we hear about a similar sense of feeling 'remarkably freer' when she hits on the notion that there are cultural differences which account for some of her problems about assessment.

Finally it should be noted that there are indications in all chapters, in the light of what the writers are discovering, of the need to offer some rather different elements in the pre- and post-registration education in these professions. There is clearly a need to lead both new and experienced professionals to take account of the primacy of practice and all that follows from learning from and through practice in the way that other writers have. Crissi's and Sheila's chapters show this in detail. Judith also makes the strong point that most health care professionals receive little training in how to teach let alone how to assess when they move from professional health care practice to professional education.

As will already be clear, many strong emotions and personal responses lie behind the revelation of these themes, and it is to these that we must turn briefly in order to register properly the overall impact of them, since they constitute a theme in their own right.

Feelings

Feelings are often the first manifestation of something slightly unusual about a professional's practice. The old traditions of calm detachment, much valued by many professionals, still govern professional behaviour under routine situations, but when this breaks down it is one sign that this piece of practice needs to be attended to carefully. Such attention to personal feeling is therefore not for selfish and/or therapeutic reasons. In art, to summarise what Joyce's hero says in *Portrait of the Artist as a Young Man*, the centre of emotional gravity needs to be equi-distant from the artist and the audience. The narrative is no longer purely personal. The personality of the artist passes into it but becomes refined and impersonalised through subsequent drafts until the writing becomes transformed into a public work. There is a strong sense that this is how it has been for our contributors.

Throughout this collection it is very clear that the chief feelings at the start of most chapters are negative ones induced by failures of various kinds to recognise and work both on and with the problematic nature of practice, or at least a particular piece of it. It is true that writers were asked to begin with a critical incident that crystallised an issue or problem in their practice (see above, p. 71), but it was indicated that this might be one which surprised, pleased, worried, angered, excited or amused. Perhaps the more negative feelings are the more memorable or the more emphatic. Certainly, anyway, both Crissi's and Sheila's chapter are characteristic here.

Sheila's emotions are of anger, turmoil, panic, agitation. Her anger recurs, spilling out again several pages into the chapter, but is gradually controlled by the force of her thinking. She admits to being concerned (and apparently horrified) that her 'reactions, verbal and non verbal, were negative and aggressive', and that her behaviour was not what she would have chosen. Significantly, once she starts to generate questions about her practice, those about her feelings come at the end of her list. Finally, in recognising that she was angry for many reasons, she puts her anger down to a reaction to the complexity of practice and then begins to accept and cope with it.

Crissi's feelings during her critical incident and the critical meeting, and the chart of the progress of those emotions are central themes in her chapter. During her chapter we see her fighting to understand them and the dilemmas of practice, and how she comes to make sense of them in terms of her personal background.

Other chapters manifest the significance of strong feelings too. Judith's main feelings of anxiety are what drive her to investigate and finally come to accept the messiness of assessment, and she notes along the way that a sense of defensiveness got in the way of accepting new ideas. Richard is frustrated with himself as well as the system, but he notes whilst being aware that it is normally not considered 'right' for professionals to talk of their feelings, that what prompts him to further reflection *is* his feeling of unease and deep sense of inner dissatisfaction – and at one point his realisation of his 'obscene enthusiasm'. He, like most writers, is also sensitive to the feelings of others. Rosemary's emotions are a mixture of dismay, disbelief and consternation as well as righteous indignation and frustration, at the malaise inherent in taking for granted the surface of practice rather than probing, understanding and working on its problematic nature, which she believes in.

In all the chapters, then, we are privileged to see the usually hidden struggle of professionals working their way from deep private emotions to new and broader-based understanding. All writers manage to control and reconsider their feelings as a result of reflecting on their practice, and all come to distance themselves somewhat from their early reactions and seem by the end of their chapters to be in more positive mood. In this way the collection probably strikes very strong chords with professionals who read it.

The writer and the reader

All the writers too are aware of issues related to their role as writers and the perspectives of the reader. Because they were not writing to any formula and not under the restraint of any model (except Clive who chose to be), the writers had to evolve their own structure, approach and style. Sheila is sharply aware of how little she had to guide her, but also of how that led her to evolve her own style. It strikes her forcefully that there is a parallel here between finding your own way of practising and your own way of writing about it, and that this involves each writer/practitioner having a style which is distinctive and individual (particular) and yet is 'embedded within a tradition'. And so it is clearly important to attend to these matters as we read. Rosemary, too, speaks of her awareness of picking words like 'acutely' and the difficulty of writing about the incident chronologically when one's thoughts resemble the tumbling of lottery numbers. Richard suggests that his interest in his incident may differ from the reader's and that the reader may want to 'flip on' to something of greater interest. Sheila draws our attention to the fact that once she had written her incident down more questions emerged, and that writing allows us to capture our more complex thinking and then to review and refine it. She says clearly that the action of writing about the practical incident has enabled her to see aspects of her practice which she had not been aware of before.

Most writers address the reader directly, and this too is a natural consequence of adopting the autobiographical form. It means that our contributors were well aware of their audience and of the likelihood of contrasting interpretations of their actions, thoughts and words, particularly in the values-based arena of professional practice and the exercise of professional judgement. Some do this more overtly than others. Judith, for example, finds the need to develop a clear relationship with her reader from the very beginning of her chapter. She says that she hopes 'to illustrate the process of reflection so that you can draw on it to critique your own experience with assessment', adds later 'the material is presented for your learning', and leaves her very last words for the reader too. She is acutely aware of the reader and comes to a new view about the reader's role as she talks about her changing view of her role as writer. Dropping the role of expert on assessment and her expectations that the literature will equip her with answers, and dispensing at the same time with the consequent belief that the reader will in turn be seeking definitive answers from her, she recognises that her expertise lies in understanding her own dilemmas and in helping the reader to do the same.

Richard too talks directly and explicitly to the reader, saying 'you will have your own views as to what was right or wrong'. Pointing up the reader's distance from and lack of personal responsibility for both professional judgement and action, he highlights how easy this makes it for the reader to think clearly as compared with how it feels for him inside the complexities of practice. He says that while the reader will see all the faults and all the solutions endemic in his incident, 'for me this remained a real dilemma'. And even Crissi, who seems less aware of her reader than some contributors, nevertheless seems to look up and focus specially on her audience in a farewell message at the end of her chapter. One of her problems, she tells us, is finishing off a piece of work like this. Is it perhaps instructive that she manages to do so here when, eventually, she addresses the reader directly?

Artistry in presentation: style, texture, tone and imagery

It is perhaps surprising, given the ample evidence of the artistry of these writers in their practice as it comes through their writing, that although, as we shall see, the imagery used is often drawn from the arts, and there is conscious artistry in their presentation, there is little overt reference to artistry in their practice, except in Clive's work where some striking points are made about professional practice as art. Perhaps, however, the words he quotes from Florence Nightingale still speak for all.

By attending a little more closely to the voices of our contributors, however, we can unravel the artistry in their presentations. Indeed, the unity of this collection and the importance of the commonalities to be found in it (as described above) is further contributed to and emphasised by our sense of the varied and different voices within it. This is not simply a group of professionals speaking 'with one voice'. Rather it is a chorus of individuals singing the same themes with different parts. And it is their written style which itself (rather like the body language of a speaker whom we can see) offers us insights into their individual character and to which as readers we relate. This is of course important from the point of view of how we read and respond to what they have to say, since we learn their stories through their own words and expressions and our response to their story is governed by our response to them or to what we are permitted or able to see beyond them.

Novelists often adopt the autobiographical point of view to convey their story, like Charles Dickens in *Great Expectations,* the first words of which are: 'My father's name being Pirrip, and my Christian name being Philip, my infant tongue could make nothing larger or more explicit than Pip. So, I called myself Pip, and came to be called Pip', or like Herman Melville in *Moby Dick*, which begins with a simple but effective reaching out to the reader in the words: 'Call me Ishmael'. Such writers know that it is vital from the beginning to engage the reader's interest in and sympathy for the main character since readers will judge how to respond to the story they are being told in the light of what they think of the teller. It is a mark of considerable artistry in the novelist to enable the reader to see *beyond* what the teller himself can see. Most of our contributors have been brave in allowing us to see and hear thoughts and ideas which later they learn to see differently, and in several chapters we, the readers, gain insight before the writer arrives at his or hers. Here they have exercised artistic control in not expunging these things in order that they themselves should appear in a better light.

But it is by the very style or texture of each chapter that the individual's stamp is put on the story. By style here then is meant the control over sentence shape and structure and the idiosyncratic phrases or descriptions and how the texture of the sentences corresponds to the content. For example, Sheila's agitation as it accompanies the speed of sudden new ideas or queries is conveyed by paragraphs of short, staccato sentences all couched as questions and culminates in a new sub-heading 'What to do?' Then she says it 'all happened in the space of a minute'. Here she almost offers us a 'stream of consciousness' approach to her tumbling thoughts (the capturing in sound and content of the untidy reactions as they come into the mind). A similar process of conveying via the sentence structure the sound of the tumbling of emotions can also be found in Crissi's work. Equally significant, though quite different, are the even tenor of Richard's reflections as he recognises with scrupulous fairness at whose door some of the problems of his practice must be placed (achieved by even length sentences and an even tone of voice together with lack of emphasis or emphatic words). And the strong sense of economy and control in Rosemary's sentences and chapter structure are in remarkable parallel to the issues of control about which she speaks.

In the use of imagery too perhaps the individuality of the writers is most striking. And the occurrence of such imagery is also noteworthy. In all the case studies imagery most often accompanies and captures (and therefore points up for the reader) moments of drama and of insight and implies accompanying emotions. Indeed, images, particularly metaphors and similes, are often a way of conveying in vivid detail ideas combined with emotion of a kind that could not be fully expressed in more prosaic terms. The insights that come to the writers through their practice and that are expressed via such images are often ideas that they knew before, but which they are only at that moment, with a sudden jolt, making their own. It is here that their learning is most evident.

It is metaphor with its sudden vividness of describing one thing in terms of another that conveys this sudden striking of new understanding, where similes offer a more slowly considered and constructed comparison using 'as' or 'like'. Thus Clive's iceberg image (reinforced by reference to hidden world and private realm) accompanies and crystallises his understanding about the artistry of practice. And vividly Judith sums up her impatience with the essential unfairness and ungovernable chanciness of assessment (and the impossibility of 'getting it right' for all students and of standardising all markers) by likening it all to playing Russian Roulette. Other striking metaphors include: Crissi's capturing of the negative and positive elements in her personality and practice in terms of electricity; Richard's consideration of personal and professional involvements in terms of boundaries; Rosemary's description of the disempowerment of nurses and the removal of their humanity in terms of their being puppets (which she reinforces later by using the words 'infanticise' and 'depersonalise'); Clive's many arts-based images of harmony, balance, and wooden (and later smooth) performance; and Judith's need for 'an assessment security blanket' in the face of the political tide of accountability and her description with its accompanying sense of distaste of how she 'traded the evaluation of professional competence ... for reproducible discrimination of technical merit'. And we should remember as we think about all this, Michael Golby's comment that metaphors are of greatest interest at the point where the comparison they are making actually breaks down (Golby, 1993).

By contrast, striking similes, which draw our attention to more considered descriptions and should therefore be noted for this reason, are fewer, but include Clive's likening of reflection-in-action (the knowledge a health care professional can have of the whole self of the patient with whom he or she is working) to an artist who has developed the expertise to know simply and precisely what shade of colour to use. Thus, through this image he comes to an under-standing of the inextricable relationship between artistry in practice and professional judgement. Judith thoughtfully explores problems implicit in marking by likening it to 'pot emptying or filling', where she uses a noticeably prosaic and boring activity and object – 'pot' being the most basic term for a vessel. And in another domestic image, which repays detailed exploration, she likens learning to assess to learning to be a parent.

It now remains to look in detail at a matter that was perhaps of greater interest to us as editors than to our writers, which is why we have placed the next set of comments in a separate chapter.

References

Fish, D. *Appreciating Practice in the Caring Professions: Re-focusing Professional Development and Practitioner Research.* Butterworth–Heinemann. In press.

Golby, M. (1993). *Case Study as Educational Research.* Fair Way Publications.

Stake, R. (1995). *The Art of Case Study Research.* Sage Publications.

Chapter 13

The centrality of professional judgement in understanding professional practice

Introduction

It is finding words like 'responsibility', 'judgement', 'argument', 'justification' and 'dilemma' in all the chapters across the collection which alerts the reader to the moral seriousness of the writing, and which points up the central thrust behind it as a shared concern about exercising judgement in professional settings. Indeed, any professional practitioner setting out to offer and reflect upon an autobiographical incident from any aspect of professional practice is, we think, likely to come sooner or later to recognise in it the judgements he or she made and to be brought to review them. Part of what we have to offer in this chapter, as a result of appreciating our contributors' practices, are some ways of making more general meanings out of these judgements which might also provide a framework to help professionals in conducting serious reflection on their own practice.

Because we believe professional judgement to be at the heart of professional practice, and when successful to be invisible, even elusive, we have chosen to focus this chapter exclusively on developing our understanding of it by reference to the practice that has been shared with us and some theoretical perspectives which have helped us. We shall of course consider both practice and theory in a properly critical light.

In so doing, however, we are aware that we are moving away from a general critical appreciation of the texts towards an interpretation of a theme that interests us (and which thus leans more towards 'interpretation' than towards a simple 'pointing up' of what is there). We are also turning gradually away from a focus upon the text itself to a consideration of matters raised by the text. We believe that this activity is legitimately covered by the term 'critical appreciation' only so long as the text figures in the processes. Towards the end of this chapter, therefore, we shall go well beyond critical appreciation and engage in an examination of professional judgement as a concept which, in Clive's terms, 'needs to be better understood' in its own right. We also hope to show why we believe that the words, 'reflection on practice', 'appreciation' (of the practical situation and of the way we present it), 'deliberation' (about the issues faced in practice), and 'judgement' (about the issues and the action they precipitate) encapsulate the heart of the processes in which professionals have to engage in order to understand better and ultimately improve their professional work.

We believe that there are a number of different kinds of judgement made during and about professional practice, and that the term 'professional judgement' means something more complicated than 'every kind of judgement made by a professional'. We are, however, deliberately taking a very broad view of judgement at the beginning of this chapter, in order not to foreclose on some piece of practice reported by our writers but which they do not describe as *professional* judgement, and in order to be sure that we take full account of all those matters of judgement endemic to their practice. We also note in passing that in the medical world, as Richard pointed out in our final meeting, it is assumed and thought to be natural that there may be conflicting professional judgements, which is why obtaining a 'second opinion' is an acceptable process.

With this broad approach in mind, then, we turn first to look, in the first section of this chapter, at the contributors' practice as reported in their writings, before turning in the second section to considering some theoretical perspectives and some deliberations about the issues raised by both theory and practice. We shall then consider what meaning we can make of professional judgement and how it might help our understanding of our contributors' writing.

Locating judgement in practical settings

Appreciating the invisible heart of practice

We have already noted that each of the chapters in Part Two is a description of each contributor's journey in the development of understanding about judgement. We have noted, too, the heavy burden of pressures on professionals to move to speedy action and to be experts in situations of great uncertainty. It is hardly surprising therefore that they themselves are not always clear about how they came to their judgements (what thinking processes they used and what they drew upon to help), nor are they able to describe the kinds of judgement (the nature of the judgements) they came to. In some cases, feelings get in the way of clarity, sometimes memory has not captured all the details, and occasionally formal theory itself blocks out action, or personal theories (which later turn out to be inaccurate) can misdirect the final judgement or decision.

But we, the readers, can say some things about judgement as it is presented in each of the chapters, and which draws upon but goes beyond what the writers themselves are fully able to articulate. This is because they describe the artistry of their practice in consciously shaped narrative which acknowledges its complexity. This means that the power of their writing conveys more than appears on the surface of the words used, and eloquently reveals some of their deeper (tacit), unrecognised levels of personal theories (beliefs, assumptions, values) that lie under their practice. And this in turn enables the reader who looks with critical appreciation to see something more than the writers themselves can articulate. Where the work focuses on that most ineffable of elements, professional judgement (which is often at once fleetingly made and yet based upon profound moral issues), critical appreciation, which senses the more subtle of nuances, is uniquely equipped to attend to what is being said and therefore to learn from it. To this end we now offer the final part of our critical appreciation of their writing.

The individual journeys in developing judgement

Rosemary

Rosemary began her work by looking at the professional judgements made by other health care professionals rather than at her own. These judgements were about her father's health care needs and even about how those professionals should relate to her parents and herself. She characterises them as routine and unthinking, and we can see that they appear not to have been made on the basis of any kind of thought, but rather to be at the level of knee-jerk reactions. By contrast, Rosemary faces and copes with her own immediate reactions and in a more deliberative way makes some important judgements of her own, deciding it wiser (having weighed up the complex pros and cons of professional duties and personal circumstances) not to raise these matters in protest at a professional level and not to import her views and feelings about the incident into her professional teaching arena. We note that, interestingly, the judgement here is that it is better to *refrain* from acting. This, of course, leaves no empirical evidence on the surface of practice either that such a judgement has been made or of the processes involved, yet the judgement is clearly a professional one since complex and contestable issues have been weighed up and more than the professional's own interests have been considered. This is a good example then of the invisibility of professional judgement, which in turn makes it so hard to study.

We are privy to the agonising involved for Rosemary in her decision-making, and quickly see how it contrasts with the reported rather careless, apparently uncaring and clearly unconsidered ("You wanted to see me did you?") speech the nurse made at her father's bedside. Indeed, it is this very contrast that leads us to interpret the nurse's words as unreflective. It might of course have been that she felt threatened, and was reacting accordingly. (This is a point that Rosemary says did not occur to her.) However, even then, 'reacting' is the word – and that is no way to describe a 'professional' judgement. As Rosemary said on reading this paragraph, a qualified nurse ought to expect to recognise or even anticipate relatives' anxieties.

It thus begins to seem that we are seeing here two very different sorts of judgement. Rosemary herself does not, however, comment on these matters in terms of professional judgement. She said afterwards that this was a conscious choice in order not to seem 'text-bookish' and because it "wasn't for me to make judgements since I was involved". In some ways, her demonstration of the contrast without an accompanying critical commentary about 'judgement' draws the reader more powerfully to come to those conclusions for him or herself, and renders the conclusions more palatable.

In fact, Rosemary's only direct comment about professional judgement comes near the end of her chapter when she shows how she values what can be learnt through reflection, and how she usefully distinguishes at the same time between technically effective and ethically enlightened actions and by implication the differing judgements that have led to them. (She says: 'increased understanding gained through reflection and critical enquiry [can] enhance our professional judgement of what might not only be "technically effective action" but also "ethically enlightened action"'.)

Crissi

By contrast to Rosemary's work, and in a courageous disclosure of actions and feelings which the reader recognises as not unfamiliar, Crissi shows how (fanned by a terrible sense of frustration in the face of the incompatible tensions of her situation as she perceives it) her emotions repeatedly affect her to the point where it is hard to make sound, clear-cut judgements. In some cases, like Rosemary, she may have made a decision not to disclose her own thoughts and feelings. This happens both in the meeting she describes as her critical meeting and in the previous critical incident with her post-registration newly appointed practitioners. Yet it is not entirely certain whether this was a clear-cut judgement or the result of being overwhelmed by the dilemmas that seem to surround her so that she could not collect together all the details on which to come to a judgement or produce an articulate, thought-through response.

Here emerge two further general problems which arise while studying professional judgement. One is that it is hard for any bystander to distinguish between a judgement which leads to refraining from action and a difficulty in coming to a judgement which leads to non-action. The other is that it is perhaps in retrospect rather than at the time that we can rationalise about our judgements and render them more deliberative. In our final meeting Crissi did say that having made her decisions she then often has doubts about them, which take a toll of her morale. She shows in her writing that she often sees herself in a no-win situation and that this can sometimes lead to poor decision-making and reluctant action (even to the point where she cannot cope with partings). At one point, however, instead of exercising control over her overt reactions, she gives vent to her personal feelings in public. And again there is some uncertainty (for the reader and perhaps for Crissi too) about whether this was an emotional reaction or a deliberate change of plan, or something of both. In any case, this is itself a common experience and the reader certainly responds to it as such, and again is brought to think more about the deliberate and deliberative nature of professional judgement.

We see too, in the twists and turns of Crissi's attempt to sort out her problems, that personal theories can misdirect decision-making and action. And somehow we know that in our own practice we the reader too are culpable in this from time to time. However, although she does not say so, both by her refusal to allow herself to come out with a knee-jerk reaction in meetings, and by her very act of exploring these matters in a public arena, Crissi also demonstrates a bold commitment to reflection and to exploring professional judgement. And because she has established a strong relationship with us as readers, we believe that her honesty and determination will enable her in future to come to clearer judgements by more reflective means.

Richard

From inside his particularly delicate arena of practice in palliative care, Richard, despite his long experience and obvious expertise, identifies four dilemmas that he faced during the incidents that made up his story and which demanded quick judgements from him in the heat of practice. And he also, with great courage and humility, quickly places himself beneath the reader's critical scrutiny. (He says: 'How one's own agenda can muddy the waters' and, directly to the reader: 'You will have your own views as to what was right or wrong.')

As he permits us, then, to see into these judgements from his own standpoint and later, through his eyes, to see the possible perceptions of others involved, we become aware that there are different kinds of judgement being operated here.

First, he judges it right (in a quickly weighed up response to a situation in which he has been before and which can be tricky) to become involved, at the request of a friend, with a dying patient for whom he has no technical responsibility. Here, he knows the risks and takes a deliberate if not deliberative decision, behind which we certainly sense a moral imperative. He then correctly insists on a formal referral from the consultant, and on the basis of this enters the action.

A little later, and acting under the pressures of time and the need to relieve pain for another human being at a weekend where the normal GP was not available, he judges it right to intervene and alter the treatment (in an area in which, although he does not say so, he is after all a very significant expert). The even tone of his writing here itself reassures us that this was not a lightly made judgement either. Matters were weighed up and immediate compassion for the patient rather than medical protocol won the day. No more than that can be expected in the cut and thrust of practice. But the pay off is an irritated GP who was clearly not working to the same agenda as Richard. Richard was clearly hoping to avoid this possibility, while we the reader tend to see it as almost inevitable. Such is the privilege of the onlooker who proverbially sees most of the game.

Becoming irritated himself, Richard sees this problem as being the result of his having stepped beyond the bounds of practice, obtruded his expertise where it was unwelcome, and antagonised a key player in the palliative care arena and for the individual patient. We sense that, as he said when he read this paragraph, he anticipated the problems but acted none the less in the misguided hope that "it would all turn out OK!" (He characterises this in our final meeting as "a rare but bad mistake" – unfairly, we believe, being over self-critical.) As a result, we can, through his writing, hear his tone of voice on the telephone, no doubt revealing his own feelings and compounding the problem by putting in jeopardy a future relationship with the GP which may bode ill for other patients. Here, then, is a new situation, a new dilemma. What Richard does in response to the GP's angry call is not based upon a judgement but (understandably) rather is a reaction that comes out of a potent mixture of frustrated feelings and thoughts, which are the more sharp for being partly self-critical, and partly righteous indignation. It adds piquancy that we seem to see this at the time while Richard portrays himself as seeing it only afterwards.

His fourth dilemma – whether to visit the patient again when called in later – is quickly resolved positively and its resolution is accompanied by his strikingly described 'obscene enthusiasm'. There is an impression that there was little weighing up of this judgement either, yet *here* we surely regard that as a positive response in the circumstances (here is a reactive decision which, despite the unadmirable emotions that accompanied it, was clearly a morally right one). And Richard's reaction when the patient finally (and inevitably) dies but at least dies peacefully, is a feeling of relief that his judgement was correct.

We have been privileged here to see behind the scenes to the movingly human worries about these dilemmas and judgements, which are shared with us without defensiveness or self-justification and in penitence that more was not achieved. But of course there are no solutions to these dilemmas – there is only the trying. As Tripp says, ' there are always competing interests and values' and so it is 'seldom if ever possible to get everything entirely right in one instance let alone all the time' (Tripp, 1993, p. 54). And there are the new resolutions for future practice that Richard lists at the end of his chapter. These, as we learnt from him after the chapter was finished, worked out well. He said then: "The opportunities occurred which I have eagerly grasped *because* of the incident." Thus, what he has really gained from all this is not a set of highly specific resolutions and recommendations, which themselves would be likely to be inoperable in some contexts, but rather a confirmation (in the face of all the expectations and assumptions that burden medical experts in terms of the judgements they are expected to deliver) that professional judgement is not an absolute and never can be and that acceptance of this can open up new ways of working.

Sheila

Sheila, in her response to the student's cry for help, also makes a number of judgements, several of which she later reverses or sees as misdirected. She also helps us further to distinguish between several different kinds of judgement.

Her first example of making a judgement is in the heat of practice, when the student asks her for help at an inopportune moment. Sheila's 'What to do?', and 'I needed to resolve this dilemma decisively and quickly' capture perfectly the feeling of panic and pressure to act, and characterise the hasty decision-making that follows an unreflective judgement (a judgement in which a decision is reached almost as a knee-jerk reaction). As she says: 'in the midst of all these thoughts and feelings I had to make some speedy decisions', and later, 'something had to be done'.

As is almost inevitable, in this kind of reactive judgement, later reflection leads Sheila to recognise its inadequacy. She says 'I had failed to solve the problem for her', and she begins to sense that she had not deliberated long enough nor actually faced her uncertainty about what the problem really consisted of. She says: 'was Mary not working hard enough or was she experiencing other kinds of difficulties?' She had relied on past knowledge of the student and assumed that it was the first of these two. She also recognises that she was not confident enough (about Mary or about research perhaps) to say that Mary's problems had great potential for her learning, and admits with some shame that she would have liked to believe that hard work would solve Mary's problems, admitting 'why I thought this way reveals much about myself and my practice'. At this point she comes to a major insight that part of the problem stems from her own complex values, beliefs and theories about the research process and adult learning, thus recognising the influence on judgement of these things. By unearthing these beliefs and values, Sheila was uncovering the potential for new and possibly better judgement and new action, this time perhaps to be based upon a more deliberative process. She notes that she was 'surprised and challenged to discover the differences between what I thought I believed and what my actions reveal about my beliefs'. She adds, 'At the same time it is exciting as I see the potential to alter how I respond and behave in future.'

Thus she demonstrates, as have other contributors, that it is from the midst of real dilemmas with which one struggles that professional judgements are called for. She says, 'I ... struggled ... not knowing how to do the best thing for the student.' (Here the focus of the problem has changed from how to find a speedy answer to how to do the *best* for the learner, and this, on any definition is therefore centrally about professional judgement.) In a final attempt to distance herself from the need to make a judgement, she then adds: 'I considered that perhaps I did not have to hand the theoretical knowledge (empirical knowledge) needed in that situation to make the "right" professional judgement'. She then questions whether there is such a thing as the required theoretical knowledge to help the judgement. 'Formal theories about research and learning have their place but the incident highlighted the complexity and uncertainty of practice. Formal theories are not very helpful in guiding one through the uncertainties of practice.' She then admits that instead she tried to rely on past experience and intuition. She says later: 'What would have been the right thing to do? The question is: right for whom, and why? Clearly the answer to this lies at the heart of my learning from the incident.' And so she recognises the need for professionals to think further about judgement and recognise the influences which impinge on it. These she characterised in our final discussion as the influences of her personal and professional goals, her student's goals, her institution's goals and those of her profession and of research. It may be that in the consideration of different goals there are different kinds of judgement.

Judith

Judith sites her critical incident in an aspect of educational practice which is fraught with problems about judgement. Assessment is often treated in the public arena as if it were a simple technical matter requiring little more than the carrying out of routine procedures (which can temporarily resolve dilemmas but cannot ultimately solve them), whilst in fact it often calls for complex professional judgement. Judith, who shows herself as coming from a positivistic background, also begins by expecting to apply some simple structure to her writing and to discover some simple solutions to her on-going puzzles about assessment. Her chapter therefore shares some of her frustrations and her decision-making along a journey from certainty to uncertainty, from unrecognised values to new awareness of the role values play in professional judgements, and from a simple bureaucratic vision of assessment to a complex educational one.

She begins by stating her most strongly held value, which she also repeats later – that judgements should be 'fair' – and by implication that they should be educational. She had experienced unfairness as a learner herself and had (without realising it) virtually recognised *at that stage* that assessment is frequently rather less about education and rather more about the need to administer politically motivated procedures. (She actually said in the final discussion, 'I'm not sure that I've recognised that even now'.) She had therefore collected but not assembled into a whole the evidence that assessment is bound to suffer from the tension between being a bureaucratic tool and an educational facility, and that a consequent tension occurs because judgements made during assessment are often torn between being about rough and ready categorisation (simple technical judgements) and an educational response to the learner's particular needs (a judgement where various problems are weighed and dilemmas are essentially insoluble, being value-based and inherently problematic).

Along her journey, Judith comes to see the tensions between the art and the science (or technology) of assessment, and to recognise its reductionist trends. She does not, however, quite come to the recognition that in wishing to go beyond the technical rational approach, she will become involved in making the kind of complex judgements about assessment that are unable to be easily managed bureaucratically. But she usefully calls our attention to the invisibility of good professional judgement ('most of the placement activities passed uneventfully'). And she raises the important issue about how one learns to make good (professional) judgements ('I was unsure how to acquire the ability to make those judgements').

She half recognises in the different judgements made of a student's performance by different people that personal values, beliefs and assumptions are central issues. And she raises issues about how professional judgements are validated, since there are some bad reasons for giving marks (particularly in our present quality control climate). She then shows that whilst she can confidently discriminate between students in terms of professional skills and technical competence, she cannot assess the artistry of practice. Thus confidently being able to justify the mark allocated for a piece of work can only be at the expense of not assessing capacities such as professional attitudes and critical thinking. In other words (although she does not say so), the administrative purpose (to discriminate between students – for whatever good reason) is incompatible with the educational purpose of assessment (to recognise, reward and give feedback on educational processes).

It is also interesting to see that as Judith wrestles further with assessment she faces (as do we all) the pressure to see it in its technical terms because these are easier to justify. Thus, in her agonising she never quite reiterates that early insight, never quite recognises that assessment is always notional, inaccurate, rough and ready, and (in its formal role) never really serves a purely educational end. Yet, somehow out of her struggle she enables us to see that where the problem of assessment is conceived of as technical (administrative, discriminatory), simplistic technical judgements will be brought up to it, but where it is conceived of as educational and problematic, it will demand more complex and problematic judgements.

Towards the end of her chapter she raises issues about the relationship between clinical and medical reasoning and judgement and assumes that there is a learnable pattern of making judgements. We shall take up this issue in a later section of this chapter.

Clive

Clive too chooses a particularly delicate (and therefore highly appropriate) aspect of professional practice – that of the place of touch in health care practice – as a 'vehicle' to develop his understanding 'of how we exercise our judgement in a professional caring relationship'. He is the writer most directly concerned with judgement (which he mainly refers to broadly as judgement rather than 'professional judgement'). This may be what leads to his use of rather technical rational terms in relation to judgement. He talks throughout his chapter of 'skilled judgement' and of 'exercising judgement'. Although he later says that he is going to question practitioners (during some tape-recorded sessions on the value of the group he is working with) on whether they had refined their knowledge of how they used *professional* judgement, he does not distinguish it from the broader term.

Later he notes that the literature does not 'fit', that our practice does not fit existing written knowledge, and that perhaps this is why 'we need to develop our professional judgement' and 'learn to rely on ourselves'. But when he gives rein to his interest in the artistry of practice he raises questions about judgement that are unique to his chapter, and he places judgement unequivocally in the realm of the artistry of practice. (But in returning to use the broader term 'skilled judgement' at this point, however, he somewhat reduces the impact of this idea.) For example, he notes that on first re-entering the practice setting he found his artistry cramped by deliberation and that his judgement appeared 'to be based on a degree of trial and error', but that as his practice increased his judgement became proficient. When this happened he 'felt in tune', and concludes that harmony is the backcloth to exercising professional judgement.

Clive then expands these ideas about judgement (he again drops the adjective 'professional') in terms of imagery drawn from the arts but also with his earlier notions of trial and error lurking behind the words. He sees skilled judgement as an artistic perform-ance and likens judgements in health care to those made by actors, dancers and painters who must rehearse, and whose judgements are a result of hours of practice (practical experience). Relating this to his own and his practitioners' work, he talks of becoming clear about the basis on which judgement was made about which intervention to use with patients. Such judgement he describes as being made on the basis of 'knowing the patient' well (having a developed understanding of how patients displayed agitation, restlessness, distress) and knowing intuitively their needs. Here he implies that there is more to artistry than skills, but does not say quite what. He does, usefully in our view, distinguish between the technical rationality of evidence-based or research-based practice and clinical effectiveness on the one hand and what he calls the 'skills' of professional judgement on the other, saying that judge-ment will remain misunderstood if we neglect our understanding of artistry or of skilled expert practice, and concludes that given the complexities of exercising judgement, more work is needed to understand it (and we would add, more work by practitioners to understand their own professional judgements). Thinking deeply in this way about practice, he argues, encourages people to explore it, and question a whole range of issues. Understanding the use of professional judgement, he says, is complex and involves profes-sionals in exploring the artistry of their skilled practice.

The collection as a whole

What can we say so far then about professional judgement from the collection as a whole?

We can say that story telling (and particularly the telling and exploring of autobiographical incidents) is a help in understanding something of the complexity of the whole picture of an episode of practice. And seeing the operation of judgement in its complex and messy practical setting in turn helps us to do justice to its complexity. For the writers there seems much to be gained by looking back on their judgements and even, in some cases, in using retrospective deliberation to render intuitive or reactive judgements rather more 'professional'. The reader, hearing the voices of the practitioners, meeting them *through* the text and learning through this about their values and beliefs, assumptions and theories, as well as about the content of their chapters and their understanding of what is involved in 'judgement', is enabled to think critically about what they have to say – both individually and across the collection.

Since we have been offered across the collection a wide range of judgements made in professional practical settings we can readily see that there is no real consensus in their use of the term 'judgement' and in their understanding of its processes. We can conclude from the collection that for these professionals at least the term 'judgement' is not *necessarily* the same as 'professional judgement' simply because a professional had made or taken or exercised it. We can also see that sometimes in the heat of practice a speedy judgement has to be made, but it is not the speed but the amount of weighing up that goes on at that instant that seems to render it 'professional' or otherwise. It may be that this 'weighing up' is what underlies the commonly held notion that experience helps decision-making and judgement.

Some judgements involve relatively simple choices. Some are routine or are rendered easier because their like has been met frequently. Some are reactive and are made so rapidly that they can only be made from within the professional's immediate world and shaped by his or her visions and understanding. But some are highly complex, demanding the unravelling of moral and ethical issues and being shot through with questions of value, beliefs and assumptions both at a personal and a professional level. And it seems possible in retrospect, as a result of reflection, to perceive these complexities as underlying what appeared at the time to be simple decisions. Problems which are highly complex can cause an 'ethical switch off' when they require instant decisions in everyday practice – both major ones where ethical issues are public and smaller ones where individuals are alone. Here, particularly in the second of these, there are many uncertainties. There is thus a clear need for an appropriate amount of time and space to be given to professional judgements if they are to be soundly based. There is a conflict here between the need for time and space and the current assumptions in health care that a busier practitioner is somehow being more efficient. It also raises issues about the arena in which the judgements are being made, and how the demands of immediacy in practice affect those judgements compared with what happens in the less pressurised arena outside practice.

Thus, we also see that practitioners in all areas of health care and despite their knowledge and experience, face enormous pressures from public assumptions that they should 'know' everything about the health care they practice, often without having been offered a formal learning base in their training and having little or no professional development through which to gain further help. And the public expect practitioners to 'know' the theory, and, increasingly, to explain practice and give evidence for decisions when sometimes they are based on pattern recognition, but sometimes they have only intuition, common-sense and even 'hunches' to go on.

It is certainly clear that there is much that is invisible about judgement – particularly when it is successful or when it involves a decision not to act. Here particularly we rely on the critical appreciation of their practice by practitioners to reveal these deeper layers for us, and to reveal them retrospectively. We can also see that flexibility in thinking about practice, and acceptance and control of emotion and absence of feeling threatened by the dilemmas, all make for better conditions in which judgement can be harnessed. And it seems likely that the very processes of reflection on practice via critical autobiographical incidents may help both to understand the operation of professional judgement and enable practitioners to reconsider and thus refine it (see also Fish, in press). But attitude is important here too. For example, whether practitioners accept that there will always be some mystery about professional practice and thus about professional judgement is of course dependent upon their view of professionalism and whether they see it as professional artistry or as entirely technical and rational.

Having looked at what the practice of our contributors offers us as a basis for understanding (as far as is possible) the operation of professional judgement, we now seek the wider perspectives on the issue which formal theory can provide, in order to take our thinking further, so that, equipped with this, we (and readers) can ultimately turn again to practice.

Theoretical perspectives: deliberating about professional judgement

Introduction

We are able to consider carefully what our contributors have to say in Part Two about judgement in the light of what we have learnt about the basis of their views. And we do not read their work and think about it in order to 'apply' their theories or practices to our own situation, but instead to see how they came to understand their practice which may be of some help in finding our own ways of understanding our own professional judgements.

Like the work of our colleagues in Part Two, formal theory of course has its own value base which needs to be understood in order to help us to think critically about what we read. And again, we make no simple assumptions about being able to apply this knowledge to our practice, but rather to aid our own critical thinking on the way to beginning to link our particular practice to the wider traditions of our profession.

As editors, our preferred framework for coming to grips with some of the perspectives on professional judgement offered by formal theory is to be found in the professional artistry and technical rational views of professionalism which we illustrated in detail in Chapter 3. The ideas presented in the main body of this part of the chapter are drawn from writers who are persuaded by the professional artistry view of professionalism with its notions that professional judgement is a central defining force of professionalism, that it is complex, unable totally to be expressed and in that sense enduringly mysterious. And that it is more – and deeper – than the sum of the parts of decision-making or of any particular practical 'skill'. First however, we must recognise the TR view of all this. Some brief examples are given here and the critique of them is best found in the arguments offered in Chapter 3.

For those who subscribe to the TR approach, professional judgement, as a complex phenomenon like theory, is of no interest and is treated as non-existent. It is replaced by terms like clinical decision-making or clinical reasoning, and (following the same simplistic behaviourist approach as does the competency-based approach to training and assessment), it is considered able to be analysed into component parts and taught under the broad headings of 'problem-solving' and 'thinking'. Here the clinician is treated as 'a processor of information' (Elstein and Bordage, 1979, p. 111), and the process as a form of reasoning enshrined in formulas.

Diagnostic clinical reasoning, for example, is thus seen as 'employing the strategy of generating and testing hypothetical solutions to problems, using cue acquisition and interpretation, hypothesis generation and evaluation'. This is regarded as employing strategies that are 'not necessarily optimal, because to calculate the optimal strategy may be too complex a task without aids' (Elstein and Bordage, 1979, p. 115). The assumptions here are that we shall ultimately be able to do it optimally when we have more help or knowledge. Such help is seen to be available in improved information processing and computer simulation and modelling. The central questions *then* become: how do clinicians use and weigh (a curious metaphor) information to help them come to a judgement, and how consistent are the judgements across judges, and how accurate are they (Elstein and Bordage, 1979, p. 120)? Here, practitioners are treated as if they were all alike, practice as if it were always routine, and judgement as if it were like prediction and probability. Mathematics and models of some complexity are then assumed to be appropriate to describing judgement. And comparisons between statistical prediction on the one hand and intuition on the other as a means of reaching a diagnosis, come inevitably to favour the former. (See, for example, Elstein and Bordage's dismissal of the work of Barrows *et al.*, 1978.) Such studies are deemed (by their writers) to be 'helpful to practising clinicians in that they can explicitly describe and prescribe utilisation of clinical information already available' (Elstein and Bordage, 1979, p. 125). And there is a strong sense that the more we know about how experts really think, the better we shall be able to teach others how to do it (see Hamm, 1984).

Even when the approach to clinical reasoning is much more humanistic and comes from work in a profession that is less wedded to the TR view, like the work in occupational therapy of Mattingly and Fleming (1994), there is none the less to be found in it an underlying view that schemes can be applied to clinical thinking and that the moral and ethical issues are of little significance beside simpler decision-making processes. Professional judgement is barely mentioned by them.

By comparison with all this, the literature based upon a professional artistry approach to professional practice does not dismiss but rather subsumes the TR ideas, setting them into a broader context which at once transforms them into a more complex and, we claim, a more realistic view of the human aspects of a professional's work.

We have been unable to find many examples from medicine itself which accept a PA view of professional judgement, the work of Katz (1984) on uncertainty in the work of doctors being a notable exception. Even writers like Eddy (1984) who recognise uncertainty as 'creeping into medical practice through every pore' (Eddy, 1984, p. 45), none the less seek to reduce uncertainty rather than learning to live with it. And those who attempt to tackle the ethical issues, like Candee and Puka (1984), focus on decision-making paths and analytic approaches. Our sources therefore come from the world of education and of education for the professions. We offer some ideas on professional judgement which we have found useful, then, from the work of Carr (1995), Schwab (1970) and Reid (1978) on deliberation, which is at the heart of professional judgement, and the work of Tripp (1993) and Grundy (1987) on professional judgement itself.

The work of Carr

We established in Chapter 4 that the work of professionals was close to Aristotle's notion of praxis. Following from this are a great number of things that can be said about professional judgement. The most important of these is about what Carr calls 'practical reasoning' (which enables professionals to decide what to do when faced with competing moral ideals, or moral conflicts or dilemmas). The arguments are as follows.

Since (as Carr says) for *praxis* the outcomes of practice cannot be pre-specified, there will always be needed (instead of learnt routines of decision-making which may be useful where only routine or technical questions are to be resolved) a form of reasoning in which **choice, deliberation** and **practical judgement** play a crucial role. Such reasoning is about deciding between competing and even conflicting moral ideals. This is particularly central to work in health care where practitioners may be required to decide on a course of action where there are conflicting ethical demands and where it is only possible to respect one value at the expense of another. Here it is impossible to resort to technical reasoning, which relies on calculations to determine what course of action to take. Practical reasoning is not a method for determining *how* to do something, but for deciding what ought to be done (see Carr, 1995, p. 68). Here both the ends and means are open to question and alternative means are often also means to different ethical ends.

Such deliberation is demanding. 'Good deliberation is entirely dependent on the possession of what Aristotle calls *phronesis* (practical wisdom). This is the virtue of knowing which general ethical principles to apply in a particular situation' (Carr, 1995, p. 71). It was the supreme intellectual virtue for Aristotle and an indispensable feature of practice. It allows the practitioner to see:

> the particularities of his practical situation in the light of their ethical significance and act consistently on this basis. Without practical wisdom, deliberation degenerates to an intellectual exercise. The man who lacks *phronesis* may be technically accountable but he can never be morally answerable. (Carr, 1995, p. 71)

Practical wisdom then, appears in a knowledge of what is required in a particular moral situation *and* both a willingness and the capacity to act upon this knowledge. It 'combines practical knowledge of "the good" with sound judgement about what in a particular situation would constitute an appropriate expression of this good' (Carr, 1995, p. 71). Thus good judgement is an essential element in practical wisdom. Judgement here being 'wisdom and prudence which takes account of what is morally appropriate and fitting in a particular situation' (Carr, 1995, p. 72). 'Judgement' then is the crucial capacity that links deliberation and practical wisdom to action.

However, the biggest problem here (to which Carr does not allude) is that of evidence. When such judgement has been exercised and action taken, the smooth surface of practice is unruffled and the success is invisible – rather it is only when a bad judgement has been made that there is evidence (of failure) available to an observer. This is a point we shall take up later in arguing for artistic narrative examples of professional artistry and their subsequent critical appreciation because it is these that enable us in some ways to capture and consider the 'ineffable' in life (and specifically in professional practice), and is a way of articulating and exploring the invisible but crucial basis of that practice.

We have referred in some detail here to Carr's work because of the need to do justice to his argument. We now turn to work that takes these ideas further.

The work of Schwab and Reid

Reid's work is based upon the original and seminal thinking of Schwab on deliberation, and comes from within the context of education and more particularly curriculum planning. Both writers therefore offer some further means of extending our understanding of deliberation. Schwab's basic definition of deliberation was quoted in Chapter 4, p. 68. As an introduction to the work of Reid we now offer a fuller version of Schwab's words, which though originally concerned with curriculum decisions none the less are equally applicable to professional judgement in all other fields, and which will make more sense for the reader at this stage of the book.

> Deliberation is complex and arduous. It treats both ends and means and must treat them as mutually determining one another. It must try to identify, with respect to both what facts may be relevant. It must try to ascertain the relevant facts in the concrete case. It must try to identify the desiderata in the case. It must generate alternative solutions. It must make every effort to trace the branching pathways of consequences which may flow from each alternative and affect desiderata. It must weigh alternatives and their costs and consequences against one another and choose not the right alternative, for there is no such thing, but the *best* one.

He adds later:

> Deliberation requires consideration of the widest possible alternatives if it is to be most effective. (Schwab, 1970, pp. 318–319)

Elsewhere in his work he admits that for the purpose of planning an educational curriculum it would be necessary to have many meetings, contributed to by many different experts and chaired by a neutral chairman. However, his basic ideas apply equally to professional development for the individual practitioner.

Reid takes up these ideas in his important book on curriculum planning. The following provides some vision of what would be involved in a profession where deliberation had become a tradition.

> A tradition of practical reasoning is built up through extending, elaborating and refining the criteria by which actions are to be justified, and showing how these criteria are to be weighed in practical situations. The growth of the tradition is made possible by the collation and discussion of examples of practice, by the insights of gifted individuals and the discovery of new possibilities through experimentation. The result is a formal accessible body of knowledge, not of a commonsense nature, of how to engage in effective deliberation. (Reid, 1978, p.50)

While Carr, Schwab and Reid offer educational perspectives on deliberation, the work of Tripp and Grundy offer us some perspectives on judgement itself.

The work of Tripp

Tripp probes what he calls professional judgements, but which seem to be judgements of all kinds made by professionals, rather than judgements specific to professionals. He works with practising teachers, and offers an approach to the development of the judgements which professionals make through what he calls the diagnosis of practice and via critical incidents, and he emphasises the values, theories, ideologies, habits and tendencies that underlie them. He argues that they are 'an excellent way to develop an increasing understanding of and control over professional judgement' (Tripp, 1993, p. 24). His work has helped us refine our ideas about critical incidents. He suggests that many decisions by professionals are really expert guesses and have 'more to do with reflection, interpretation, opinion and wisdom than with the mere acquisition of facts and "prescribed right answers"' (Tripp, 1993, p. 124). He provides useful language when he characterises the non-clinical setting in which professionals deliberate as the 'field of discourse', which he contrasts with the clinical setting which he characterises as the 'field of action'. This is significant in that, as we saw in the work of our contributors, different kinds of deliberation, decision-making and judgement are possible in these two differing arenas.

He also usefully suggests that judgements can be considered as practical, diagnostic, reflective or critical. Each is characterised by differing kinds of information required to make the judgement, differing questions to be asked and different personnel involved. Thus, for example, for what he calls the **practical judgement** (which he says 'is the basis of every action taken in the conduct of teaching and the majority of which is made instantly', Tripp, 1993, p. 140), the information required is procedural, and the key question is 'what should I do?' **Diagnostic judgements** seem to be more about general decisions made as part of almost any kind of work. It is in what he calls **reflective judgement** that we begin to move into the kinds of judgements which we would argue are specifically *professional* judgements. He characterises reflective judgements as personal, evaluative or justificatory. He shows that these are judgements where the professional thinks about his or her actions and judges the effects of them and weighs up alternative strategies. This, Tripp notes, involves moral deliberation. He characterises reflective judgements as 'involving the identification, description, exploration and justification of the judgements made and values implicit and espoused in practical ... decisions and their explanations' (Tripp, 1993, p. 140).

Tripp's final category is **critical judgements.** He links these unequivocally with action research, which for reasons already rehearsed (p. 65 above) we would not wish to do. He says that critical judgements involve 'both a reflective critical attitude and the gathering of diagnostic information about professional practices through more formal and interventional research strategies' (Tripp, 1993, p. 137). This involves being prepared for self-criticism of a deep kind. It is interesting that Tripp notes here that writing as a process helps in this.

The work of Grundy

Clarifying the term professional judgement

The work of Grundy shows us how beliefs about relationships between theory and practice are linked to differing world views and offers us three kinds of judgement employed by practitioners in decision-making about practice. Drawing on ideas of Habermas, Grundy highlights three systems of knowledge generation and organisation, which can shape deliberation. These are: the technical, the practical and the emancipatory. Only a brief idea of them can be given here.

The technical, practical and emancipatory systems of knowledge

Grundy shows how Habermas's 'technical approach' (Aristotle's *poesis*) is concerned with questions about what the practical worker should do on the spot. This seeks to improve outcomes by improving skills. Such an approach allows knowledge to be controlled by one group alone (within, for example, education or health) and sees success in professional practice strictly only in terms of effectiveness and efficiency. Here the view of theory is that theory directs, confirms and legitimises practice. Here the only judgement left to be operated by the practitioner is **strategic judgement** – about what to do to attain a given end. Those who follow this approach practise according to rules and use their skills to a pre-determined end. This brings with it a 'deficit view' of practitioners – an assumption that professionals are below standard – because it is based upon the idea that the system needs to be virtually foolproof to ensure that practitioners need only to follow rules in order to 'get it right' and that even the poorest practitioners will manage that much. (Ironically, of course, this penalises better practitioners by binding them to procedures that they would be capable of but which they would be well able to go beyond.) This view also has implications for curriculum design for both professional preparation and professional development courses where that which Stenhouse calls the product model (see Stenhouse, 1975) becomes the inevitable basis for what must be a version of *training*, since what a practitioner would need in this view would be skills or competencies.

By contrast, Grundy suggests that, via Habermas's 'practical approach' we can see practice as guided by choice which in turn is guided by a disposition towards what is 'good' (Aristotle's *praxis*). This involves an aspect of moral consciousness. There is greater choice here for the practitioner. The practitioner here would break rules if he or she judged it necessary for 'good'. Here the practical decisions have to be made in the actual situation. This involves what she calls 'practical judgement' which is exercised through deliberation (or reflection). According to Grundy (1987, p. 65), 'Deliberation incorporates processes of interpretation and making meaning of a situation so that appropriate action can be decided upon and taken.' All participants have equal rights in interpreting or making meaning out of a situation. The practitioner chooses action guided by personal judgement, having understood the situation. This means that practitioners are educated rather than trained. Here theory provides a guide not a direction, and curriculum planning is on the basis of what Stenhouse calls the process model (see Stenhouse, 1975). Judgement, though not a skill, is seen as being able to be developed through processes of reflection. Meaning-making in a democratic environment is vital – and is helped by writing as well as talking. Further, Grundy shows that, 'as well as knowledge arising directly through reflection upon practice, Habermas's "practical interest" encourages the development of knowledge through the bringing to consciousness of implicit theory, thus providing a more consciously rational basis for action' (Grundy, 1987, p. 77).

Grundy's third or 'emancipatory' orientation engages practitioners in the active creation of knowledge on the job. (In some senses it is perhaps a more fully developed version of Aristotle's *praxis*.) Here, significantly, the word 'critique' is taken to mean a more fundamental questioning of both theory and practice than is implied in the 'practical approach' and in the more traditional usage of the term 'critical thinking'. The locus of control for making judgements about the quality and meaningfulness of the work lie with the participants in what is seen as the learning situation and there is freedom to question accepted wisdom, recognise that things are not as they seem to be and develop a sophisticated critical consciousness where questioning leads to investigation which leads to critical insight. This authentic critique 'looks back at theory and, while trying to make meaning of it, critically examines its value for practice' (Grundy, 1987, p. 132).

This engages the practitioner in exercising **professional judgement**. Here theory is looked to for information but not for direction. This approach 'brings enlightenment concerning the real conditions of existence' (Grundy, 1987, p. 157), and transforms consciousness – enables us to see the constraints within which our practice occurs and to break out of habitual ways of seeing things and of acting. This approach (which is difficult to achieve at the best of times) is perhaps more easily achievable in a teaching/learning workplace than in the practical workplace of, say, health care. In curriculum design terms teaching and learning are regarded as problematic, the teacher is taught in a dialogue along with the student, and both theory and practice (and all means and ends) must be open to critical scrutiny. Grundy argues the 'emancipatory approach' provides for authentic learning by students as opposed to the 'co-opted agreement' which characterises other approaches (Grundy, 1987, p. 125). Here knowledge is socially constructed, the teacher recognises 'moral constraint in the extent to which student learning may be coerced' (Grundy, 1987, p. 127), and the learner can thus control the learning situation. Here dialogue is a vital means of learning, and a curriculum is not a written plan but an active process in which planning, acting and evaluating are reciprocally related. By this means, Grundy and her fellow thinkers distinguish sharply between broadly 'reproductive' and radically 'transformative' approaches to education (and practice).

But in our view this 'emancipatory' approach unfortunately reserves the term professional judgement for very rare occurrences, of a rather idealised kind, and links the whole enterprise to notions of social transformation with which those engaged in *praxis* might not wish to associate. We would therefore wish to borrow strategies from this ideal approach, seeing praxis as served by a full critical consciousness, and using the term professional judgement rather more broadly to mean being able to break out of traditional ways of seeing theory and practice, without necessarily having to subscribe to the social transformation philosophy. And we believe that this is not unreasonable, since if all theory and practice are to be considered critically and used eclectically, then so is the 'emancipatory approach' itself!

We also find Grundy's terms somewhat confusing since the words 'strategic', 'practical' and 'professional' seem, when linked to the word judgement, rather too common to carry the weight of meaning she wishes to attach to them, and since she does not seem to discriminate between them in respect of deliberation, which she seems to imply is in all of them.

Equipped then with the contributors' experience from practice, and these theoretical perspectives, we now present our own attempt to map a little more clearly the various kinds of judgement that our colleagues wrote about. Particularly we seek to provide a framework to aid the understanding of practice, and therefore for use *and for critique* by readers who want to investigate their own practice further and try to understand it better, and for those who wish to return again to our colleagues' writing in Part Two.

Making sense of professional judgement

We here attempt to describe four broad categories of professional judgement which we consider to be key points along a *continuum* from sub-professional, unconsidered response, through to highly enlightened decisions by deliberative practitioners. We have based our work on the ideas of Tripp and Grundy, but have used different terms from theirs because we found theirs internally confusing (the term 'practical judgement' being used differently by each, for example) and unmemorable. Our proposed four broad areas of judgement then, are: **intuitive judgement; strategic judgement; reflective judgement** and **deliberative judgement**. We see these as operating along a continuum. All four are utilised throughout their work by professionals. We would reserve the term 'professional judgement' for use wherever thinking like a professional is involved, which we believe could apply even to the first broad category when intuitive judgement is *considered*, retrospectively.

We shall attempt to indicate for each kind of judgement in turn the kinds of practical question endemic to it, the type of question involved, the kind of response assumed, the kind of thinking involved, the role of theory in that thinking, and the role the practitioner takes on as a result of this whole. Table 13.1 below acts as a summary of all this.

Intuitive judgement is at one end of the continuum and lies furthest away from highly deliberative activity. It concerns itself with urgent practical questions needing immediate response in the field of action. Such questions can be characterised as: "What *do* I do *now*?", and involve (or *appear* at the time to involve) a relatively simple choice, usually about how to do something and what skills to call on. There is no overt reasoning involved in the response. The practical response can be to react in a habitual or ritual way informed

Table 13.1 Making sense of professional judgement: key points on a continuum

Actual question	Type of question (kind of reasoning)	Practical response	Kind of judgement	Role of theory	Role of practitioner
What *do* I do *now*? (about skills, how to do something) A quick decision	**Practical question** (no reasoning involved)	**React in habitual way** (informed by routine or shaped by emotion or a knee-jerk reaction)	**INTUITIVE JUDGEMENT** Unreflective	**Theory not recognised** (all knowledge tacit)	**Practitioner as automaton or junior mechanic** (no refinement of practice possible. Reduces professionalism) A reactive move
What *might* I do now? (about skills and actions) A simple choice from a list	**Procedural question** (involves procedural reasoning and choice of techniques)	**Review the practical possibilities from *inside* practice uncritically** (select tactics pragmatically) Thinking is done in rough catagories	**STRATEGIC JUDGEMENT** Reflection only after the event, if at all	**Theory confirms and legitimates skills-centred practice** (some surface tacit knowledge unearthed)	**Practitioner as technician** (refinement of skills possible but a slave to ends) A forced move with no real justification

Table 13.1 (continued)

Actual question	Type of question (kind of reasoning)	Practical response	Kind of Judgement	Role of theory	Role of practitioner
What could *I* do now? (for my own sake as a professional) Decision seen as a more complex matter – a mix of skills, knowledge, capacities	**Prudential question** (involves prudential reasoning) A choice from amongst own skills, abilities, knowledge	Personal judgement made which takes account of professional's own skills and abilities and the complexities of the practical situation (picks way forward to please self; assumes ends fixed)	**REFLECTIVE JUDGEMENT** Reflects on actions both during and after events taking an evaluative stance and is critical (in that limited sense)	Theory enlightens practice and is enlightened by it, but focus is still on means only (not ends) and skills (more (deeper) tacit knowledge revealed)	Practitioner as independent (senior) technician (a thinking professional; refinement and development of skills-based work is a natural part of practice) A move with relative justification
What *ought* I to do now? (for the good of patients) This is moral enquiry using practical reasoning and practical wisdom	**Moral ethical question** (practical reasoning – complex choice about what to do when faced with competing moral ideals, dilemmas) Practical wisdom vital	Active practical enquiry about what should be done for the best, good of patients or clients (ethically enlightened) Take holistic view	**DELIBERATIVE JUDGEMENT** Deliberates on ends and means; has disposition to be critical, take nothing for granted, break out of habitual ways of seeing, question the accepted	Practitioner tries to make meaning of theory and practice, examines critically own moral values (uncovers espoused theories and theories-in-action)	Practitioner as enlightened professional (a professional in charge of own practice, willing and able to investigate means and ends) A move with a general justification

by routine, or shaped predominantly by emotion and understood (if at all) from within the practitioner's normal ways of seeing. At its furthest end of the continuum, this involves what are often called knee-jerk reactions – the term itself indicating that there is no thinking (no *apparent* thinking) involved. This broad area characterises unreflective judgements where the role of personal theory (which nevertheless shapes it) is not recognised, and where formal theory is treated as non-existent. Here the practitioner is adopting roles which can range from automaton to junior mechanic. Here there is no hope of the practitioner refining or improving his or her own practice at least until reason is engaged and new understandings are used to enlighten these reactions (though practitioners could of course be directed by someone else to change their practice). As a result, the work involved cannot be described as specifically 'professional' in any meaningful sense (and indeed, there are those in power who seek to place the professional in circumstances where more and more judgements of this kind only are required, in order to control their professional influence).

Strategic judgement (a term we borrow from Grundy for this category) also concerns itself with urgent practical questions, but assumes – and is interested in – a wider range of possibilities. The characteristic question here might be: "What *might* I do now?" This too is about skills and action, and is basically a procedural question, calling for a review of practical possibilities, and which harnesses technical reasoning for doing so. Here the practitioner, still working from inside his or her habitual view of practice, and thinking uncritically and in rough and ready categories about a range of possible actions and responses, selects pragmatically a set of tactics. There is no consideration at the time of how to justify the decision and consequent actions, although there *could* be reflection upon it after the event. It is at the time, therefore, a forced move with no real justification, though sometimes formal theory can be almost ritually called upon to legitimise and confirm this essentially skills-based practice.

This sounds to us essentially to be a description of what in practice is involved in evidence-based practice (at least where practice is governed by protocols and guidelines)! The practitioner here becomes (or in the case of guidelines or protocols is made into) a technician. Where reflection does occur after the event, both personal and formal theory might be drawn upon, and some tacit knowledge is likely to be unearthed. Here refinement of skills by the professional is possible where reflection is engaged. But, even at the end of the continuum nearer to enlightened professionalism, there will only be refinement of skills, the ends or goals will be accepted, and the practitioner will be a slave to them, either knowingly or without realising it if no reflection is involved.

Reflective judgement is a term Tripp uses to characterise the kind of judgement which involves the practitioner in practical reasoning. We use it to crystallise that point along our continuum where the question is focused upon practice and may need to be considered in the heat of practice but essentially calls for deeper thought. Here the practitioner recognises and engages with the complexities of practice, including skills, knowledge, attitudes and capabilities but still sees them from within his or her own settled view of professionalism. A characteristic question would be: "What could *I* do now?" The implication of the emphasis is that the practitioner is focusing upon decisions made *for his or her own sake*, and taking account of personal attributes and motivations. Here we have what are broadly prudential questions involving prudential reasoning and a choice from amongst the practitioner's own comfortable repertoire. Here an essentially personal judgement is made where the practitioner takes account of his or her own skills and personal abilities, weighs up the complexities of the practical situation as seen from within his or her settled practices, and chooses a way forward which pleases and suits him or her. But this still involves an acceptance that the ends or goals of practice are fixed. Here personal theory particularly but formal theory also, enlightens practice, but is used only to consider means and skills. Here there is some real justification for what is done. Deeper (tacit) personal theory is revealed and the practitioner becomes a more senior and even an independent technician – a thinking and thoughtful practitioner. Here refinement and development of the means of practice are a natural part of practice and can be called upon both during it and in retrospect, that is in the fields of both action and discourse.

Deliberative judgement lies at the far end of this continuum. Here, the question is a moral and ethical one, characterised in the query: "What *ought* I to do now?" Here the thrust of the question is away from the practitioner and concerns itself with the good of the client or patient. Here the whole enterprise of professional practice is seen as a form of moral enquiry, utilising practical reasoning and practical wisdom. Here the professional sees practice as involving competing moral ideals, moral conflicts and unresolvable dilemmas – as concerned with the essentially contestable. This engages practitioners in making complex choices which yield to no simple, known calculation. Here practical reasoning must be harnessed to practical wisdom (which does not have a simple relationship to age, status, or length of experience in practice). Without practical wisdom this would be a purely theoretical and intellectual exercise and have no place in the field of discourse let alone the field of action.

We believe that it may be this quality of practical wisdom together with its incalculable relationship to practical reasoning which lies at the heart of the mystery of practice and which we believe can be explored further (but never absolutely) by appreciating the artistry of practice. Here the practical response is practical enquiry about what should be done for the best or good of the patient or client. Here the professional becomes ethically enlightened and freed to question accepted wisdom in all areas, which include the aims or goals (the outcomes) of practice as well as the means (the processes). Here practice can be given a general justification. Here professionals are always prepared to recognise that things are not always as they seem, will not take anything for granted, and as a consequence (not as an objective) develop critical insight, reflection and deliberation. Thus deliberative judgements entail deliberation about the ends and the means of practice and are critical in that they involve the professional in developing the disposition to take nothing for granted and to break out of habitual and comfortable ways of seeing professional work, themselves and their own practice. Here then, professionals try to make meaning of their own theory and practice as well as of formal theory and the traditions of the profession to which they belong. This involves examining critically their own moral values and uncovering and exposing to reconsideration their espoused theories and theories-in-use. Here the professional is an enlightened practitioner – a professional in charge of his or her own professional work, thoughtful about ends and means, able and willing to investigate both, and accountable for *and* able to give an account of his or her practice.

A summary of these four points which we have crystallised on the broad continuum from mechanic to enlightened professional can be found in Table 13.1.

We suggest that all four broad kinds of judgement are utilised by professionals in the field of action and the last three in the field of discourse, and that often judgements can be best understood as somewhere along the continuum between these four – either at the time or retrospectively. The idea of a continuum allows for some judgements to fall somewhere between neighbouring points. An example of this might be a professional judgement to react quickly in order to maintain the flow of an action, to redress an imbalance or because any decision was better than none. Although the word 'reaction' suggests that this is an intuitive judgement, none the less it has been made with more thought and justification than a knee-jerk one, though of course it is possible that in retrospect the practitioner may not be sure just how far the judgement was thought out rather than reactive.

We emphatically reject the notion that these key points along the continuum are related in a simple way to different levels of professional expertise, status, age or years of experience, and we equally reject the notion that they might be found differentially in practitioners of differing lengths of service or of ability, or be found located within the novice to expert model as suggested by Benner (1984). We also have come to believe, as a result of responding to our colleagues' work, that it is possible *retrospectively* to reflect upon or deliberate about intuitive and strategic judgements made in practice, to discover them to have been of a different nature from that which we originally assumed, and to recognise only then why one came to the decision or to provide a retrospective rationalisation for it. We also believe that through retrospective reflection and deliberation we might come to see a judgement we have made as being located towards the lower end of the continuum (having considered it at the time as being higher) and that through that reflection and deliberation our judgement in future might be more enlightened. In other words, by uncovering our judgements (including those that are invisible because they involve the decision *not* to act) and reflecting upon them we believe that it is possible to develop our judgements because we understand more about them and about how we as individuals come to them. We hope that this model will both help professionals in that process and be subjected by them to further critique and refinement or new development.

References

Barrows, H. S., Feightner, J. W., Neufeld, V. R. *et al.* (1978). *Analysis of the Clinical Methods of Medical Students and Physicians.* McMaster University School of Medicine.

Benner, P. (1984). *From Novice to Expert: Excellence and Power in Clinical Nursing Practice.* Addison-Wesley.

Candee, D. and Puka, B. (1984). An analytic approach to resolving problems in medical ethics. In *Professional Judgement: a Reader in Clinical Decision Making* (J. Dowie and A. Elstein, eds.), pp. 474–487. Cambridge University Press.

Carr, W. (1995). *For Education: Towards Critical Educational Enquiry.* Open University Press.

Eddy, D. M. (1984). Variations in physician practice. In *Professional Judgement: a Reader in Clinical Decision Making* (J. Dowie and A. Elstein, eds.), pp. 45–60. Cambridge University Press.

Elstein, A. S. and Bordage, G. (1979). Psychology of clinical reasoning. In *Professional Judgement: a Reader in Clinical Decision Making* (J. Dowie and A. Elstein, eds.), pp. 10–129. Cambridge University Press.

Fish, D. *Appreciating Practice in the Caring Professions: Re-focusing Professional Development and Practitioner Research.* Butterworth–Heinemann. In press.

Grundy, S. (1987). *Curriculum: Product or Praxis?* Falmer Press.

Hamm, R. M. (1984). Clinical expertise and cognitive continuum. In *Professional Judgement: a Reader in Clinical Decision Making* (J. Dowie and A. Elstein, eds.), pp. 78–107. Cambridge University Press.

Katz, J. (1984). Why doctors don't disclose uncertainty. In *Professional Judgement: a Reader in Clinical Decision Making* (J. Dowie and A. Elstein, eds.), pp. 544–565. Cambridge University Press.

Mattingly, C. and Fleming, M. (1994). *Clinical Reasoning: Forms of Inquiry in a Therapeutic Practice.* F. A. Davis.

Reid, W. (1978). *Thinking about the Curriculum: the Nature and Treatment of Curriculum Problems.* Routledge and Kegan Paul.

Schwab, J. J. (1970). The practical: a language for curriculum. In *Joseph Schwab: Science, Curriculum and Education, Selected Essays* (I. Westbury and N. Wilkof, eds.), pp. 287–321. University of Chicago Press.

Stenhouse, L. (1975). *An Introduction to Curriculum Research and Development.* Heinemann.

Tripp, D. (1993). *Critical Incidents in Teaching: Developing Professional Judgement.* Routledge.

Chapter 14

Giving professionalism back to professionals

Introduction

This last section was written shortly after we held a final workshop with the contributors – a four-hour session where we discussed, amongst other things, a draft of Part Three, and considered in some detail what to say now the project was over. We also reviewed the project as a whole, its origins, the contributors' involvement, our own input, the processes we had all been through, and the outcomes as we now saw them. We video-recorded this discussion, and by reviewing the tape and transcribing what people said, we added further data to our project, with the bonus of seeing on video how people said what they said and how we (as well as the others) reacted.

What we hope to do then in this final section is firstly to try to say where we sense we are now. Next we will describe how we managed to get to this point, that is to describe (more fully now than we could at the outset) the process we all went through, as it has emerged in reality. Following this we will say what we believe all of this has added up to, what the outcomes are of asking a group of expert practitioners to go through a certain process. And finally, in the last chapter, we will suggest what we believe all this means, particularly for professional practice, professional education, and practitioner research.

Where are we now?

We set out by asking a group of experienced practitioners from a range of health care professions to reflect upon and deliberate in a particular way about their practice (or, at least initially, on an incident they took from their practice) and then to write about this, not just about the incident nor indeed just about their practice, and not just to reflect in some armchair way on their practice but to tell us about their reflections on their practice. What emerged (through this autobiographical approach) was a 'collection' of pieces – where the whole is greater than the sum of the parts.

And from this we believe there has emerged a set of observations concerning the current state of health care practice at the end of the twentieth century and of practitioners working within it. In summary we list these as follows.

- Professional work is a complex phenomenon, and working as a professional is a complex business. Learning to be a professional means becoming part of, sharing in, and dealing with that complexity.
- Even experienced practitioners face confusions and unresolved (possibly unresolvable) tensions, perhaps more now than ever before. Simply recognising and acknowledging this helps them enormously.
- But sadly most professionals do not have the opportunity in the course of their daily practice to look in depth at what they do routinely and to resolve its complexity.
- And the gap this leaves in the life of a professional, of never clearly understanding the basis of one's professional practice, only became apparent to our colleagues (and to us) as together we made slow (and sometimes painful) progress with them in reflection and deliberation.
- The principle value of this process to the contributors lay in them valuing themselves more, feeling more complete as professionals, and more confident in doing what they did.
- They recognised (to their surprise) that their professional actions (the decisions and judgements they made) were determined more by their own personal theory – their values, beliefs, assumptions and expectations – than by the formal theory they heard, read or had been told.
- The one exception (regarding the input into her thinking of formal theory) was a member of the group currently emersed in the academic study of education, initially through a masters

degree and now through doctoral research in the field of professional education. For her there is no distinction between formal and personal theory but a fusion of the two into one.

- All held the belief, which they could verify in their own practice, that this 'feel good' (or at least feel better) outcome was indeed cashing out in very real terms in their own work as practitioners.

- Yet at the same time they recognised that their experience of professional well-being through greater understanding of their practice was unlikely to convince their more sceptical colleagues of the value of this approach. They had had the experience and knew the outcomes of it for themselves. Others, in order to appreciate this, would have to undergo the same processes. They could not pass on their experience to others.

- They saw at the present time in their professional lives an emphasis on, and for them an overvaluing of, outcome measures which determined the success of health care, and they were left uncertain that the deliberations they had gone through would 'catch on' in the present climate.

- Yet they felt the time was ripe for a project such as they had experienced, that many practitioners 'out there' were, like them, unconvinced by the current headlong rush to improve practice through the contractual process, and sensed that there must be some other way but until now had not quite known what it might involve.

- There is an incompatibility between the way the contributors are now thinking about their practice and the (currently reinforced) view of professionalism which we characterised at the start of this book as the technical rational approach.

- While much lip service is paid to the 'artistic side' of practice and of how important it is to reflect on what we do, there is no urgency that these notions should become a crucial and necessary part of professional work.

- Equally the contributors saw a conflict between the work they had undertaken here and traditional views of research. Yet at the same time they recognised quite clearly what they had done to be legitimate research – an enquiry after meaning leading to a growing understanding of why we do what we do and thence to improve our practice.

- There was for them through the project a fundamental questioning of what an expert really is: not someone who simply knows a lot, does good work, or has practised for a long time, but someone who is capable of deep reflection – who knows how to undertake deliberation about his or her own practice, learns from the appreciation of it and recognises the worth of these activities in helping personal practice to develop.

- The contributors also recognised that this approach can apply at all levels of professional development, and should not be restricted to a particular phase of education.
- Nevertheless they saw that the approach they had been through requires support, encouragement, nurturing and valuing. It is only likely to occur within a conducive environment, in a culture which recognises and values it, and which wholeheartedly commits resources to its implementation.

How did we get here?

If these were the outcomes of this project for the contributors, what were the processes they went through in order to get there? In retrospect these are the key features of it.

- Fundamentally the process began with practice. We asked the contributors to identify an incident within their practice that they would like to spend some time considering. We were guided in this partly by our own experience, and partly by recognising the failure of much professional education which so often begins with formal theory which must then be applied to practice, which we almost intuitively knew to be false. We were also aware of Schön's notion of 'surprise', that is the sensation practitioners experience when some aspect of their practice is unusual or does not quite fit (Schön, 1983). The chosen incident, we suggested, could be a dilemma our colleagues had experienced, or perhaps some confusion in their practice. As it turned out, all of the incidents they reported reflect, as Richard put it at the final workshop, "some human situation" – or small moral crisis. We believe that this underscores an essential principle for professional education and development, namely the primacy of practice.
- All through the project we (as a group) acknowledged and valued our colleagues' incidents. This in itself was somewhat novel for

them. Incidents of the kind our colleagues presented are rarely discussed by fellow professionals. Indeed, they are likely to be the very situations we keep most quiet about either because they seem so trivial or because we would not want to admit to them!

- The contributors felt the supportive environment we provided was crucial for work of this kind. They commented warmly about our acknowledgement and valuing of their incidents, and of our support for them as colleagues. They felt legitimised professionally, that we saw their incidents as part of the hurly-burly of professional life, not something unusual let alone something about which they should be embarrassed or even ashamed. Merely hearing about other people's incidents gave them a greater sense of community, one they had never experienced before (which we feel was like, but not the same as, 'a community of scholars'). In a sense we had helped them create something more – a community of deeply thoughtful practitioners.

- They said much, too, about the importance of group work. They were unsure that they would have gone very far (if at all) into their practice on their own. And even if they had, they feared that working alone could lead to even greater self-deception. A collaborative, corporate approach was more than helpful – it was essential. Yet this needed to be, if not with like-minded people, at least with people who were prepared to attempt the process. At the final seminar, at least two of our six colleagues confessed to having been sceptical at the start.

- The contributors recognised the importance of the setting in which we held our workshops. We allowed plenty of time (two to four hours) at locations away from most of our normal workplaces. We were relaxed and informal yet focused and business-like.

- The process we went through essentially meant engaging in the articulation of thoughts – putting them into words (our own words). Group discussion was helpful of course but so too was the writing up. Thinking, speaking and writing (all different forms of articulation) were all needed. We had to think through what we were doing and uncover what we believed. We found that speaking about this helped. The contributors saw that they had two tasks in this articulation: on the one hand to recognise (and appreciate) the artistry in their practice, and on the other to present that artistry in an artistic manner. Yet if at the outset they had doubts that their practice was artistic they had even greater reservations about being able to present it (especially in writing) artistically – they did not see themselves as artists in either sense. Yet through the project they came to appreciate the art (and the artist) within them, and the writing – having to put things down in black and white – proved to be the essential discipline needed to make clear – in clarifying it for others – what precisely they were wanting to say.

- Through the project, deliberation occurred at many levels. The contributors spoke to us in metaphorical terms such as onion layers – it was like peeling one layer off only to reveal yet another, and so on. They felt they were constantly uncovering more and more issues, going deeper and further, unearthing matters which at the start they had no notion would emerge, exhuming some grisly skeletons but unearthing precious treasures too. And it was in this uncovering that their greatest insights occurred.

- A further way in which they characterised their practice was with the imagery of the iceberg – with only a small part of it showing but a great deal hidden (from themselves as well as others) which supported it. We will return to this notion later and explore it further.

- Theorising – identifying and clarifying one's personal theories – was a valuable, even crucial, part of the uncovering process. Not only this, but recognising too that an espoused theory – the basis on which one says one operates – was not necessarily the same as one's theory-in-use – the personal theory on which some observer of our practice might consider we were operating. They also recognised some dissonance between the two – that we do not always do what we say or say what we do – which helped them understand even more clearly the tensions and confusions in their professional practice.

- They recognised, as the process continued, that they were moving further and further away from their starting point – the incident that triggered their reflections. They were beginning to explore their professional practice more widely than the incident that started the process. Not only were they looking more broadly at their practice but they saw it more deeply too, not just in those practical aspects of what they were doing day in and day out but more particularly (and probably more importantly) they were exploring the very basis of their professionalism – what it was that made them work the way they did. While understanding their theoretical basis, they now asked themselves what their philosophical basis was. How consistent were they? Did they do something in one situation on the basis of a certain set of beliefs but do something quite different in another based on a different and perhaps conflicting set of beliefs?

- And as they unravelled all of this, as they peeled back the onion layers, as they explored beneath the surface of their iceberg, they began to see how these differences and distinctions had never been addressed before. They had never taken the time (never had the time, or been encouraged to take the time) to do this. Yet this dissonance was there – inside them – nagging away at them, all the time chipping away at their self-confidence. They knew they were not always being consistent but they had never, until now, known why, let alone seen this unravelling as a way forward.

- Two of the contributors reported that before the project they often found themselves in situations when, as they put it, they 'felt a fraud'. By this they meant that in carrying out a piece of practice which they knew to be appropriate they would nevertheless, if challenged, have been quite unable to give a satisfactory explanation as to why they had done what they did. In these circumstances they would often resort to using terms such as 'it was intuition' or 'a gut feeling', perhaps adding 'it comes with experience'. They recognised that such explanations, which were unsatisfactory to them and probably to their listeners, certainly did not help when they were asked to be accountable for their actions. Even more crucially they were of little help to them as teachers when attempting to pass on to learners the foundations of practice, or as examiners when being required to assess the practice of others. Now they could. Not that they would always know the basis of a particular piece of practice nor that telling someone else their theoretical basis would mean the other person's practice would change but, more importantly, they now knew a way of articulating their practice and of encouraging others to do so as well.

- The formal theory of professional practice, found in books and journals, was something of a problem for most of the contributors. (Only those who had studied education at masters level had been exposed to this through formal study.) After deliberating on their practice some found it helpful, even illuminating to read some of the literature. It made sound sense of what they were now thinking. It summed it up. For others in the group, even after the event, the theory was strangely unhelpful or lacked impact. But for most of them, it was of very limited use prior to their deliberations. (For this reason we offered our colleagues very little formal input at the start – other than the sheets we have appended to Chapter 4 – and only small amounts of theory during the workshops we had with them.) The contributors came to recognise that formal theory was not easy to apply to practice, and on occasions it conflicted with their experience. As Clive said at the final workshop: "You might know something but it does not always help you in practice."

- Most of our contributors had developed, through engaging in this process, a much greater confidence in their own thoughts regarding the basis of their professional practice. As Judith said at the final workshop: "If you're running to other authors [for support] what's to say that their view is valid just because they happen to have published it. Mine is now valid because I happen to have published it. I found that looking at my own personal history and its influence on my behaviour and attitude was a terribly, terribly important part [of the process]."

What does all this add up to?

So where does this get us? What does engaging in this project add up to? What can we conclude from our observations of our colleagues' writing (as well as our own) and their reflections on the process we have all been through?

In Chapter 11 we wrote 'the ultimate intention of this book is to free readers to conduct their own explorations of their own practice and thus to see the examples offered ... not as new knowledge to be applied to their own practice but simply as examples of reflection on practice to encourage similar yet different explorations of their own'. We believe this most strongly. In a very real sense we believe the contributors were 'freed' by engaging in the project. And we see this freeing at three levels: the practical, the theoretical and the personal. We will take each one in turn.

First at the practical level we provided certain means whereby we hoped our colleagues would engage in serious reflection upon and deliberation about their professional practice and thus gain greater insight into it.

These practical means have been described above. Fundamentally they included: recognising the primacy of practice, identifying incidents, making available printed sheets with suggested frameworks for looking at practice, using an autobiographical approach, theorising, reflecting, reflecting on reflection, crystallising and distilling the issues, peer review, input from ourselves as editors (including providing a conducive environment), colleagueship, collaboration, regular seminars and workshops, and so on, and finally offering a further critical appreciation.

So we gave the contributors the practical means for reflection and deliberation and even some of the language of deliberation which up to then they had not necessarily been aware of or recognised as being valuable in the pursuit of developing their professional practice. Moreover these were not activities which had formed part of their education up to that point, nor had they taken time (or been given leave) to engage in these practices. Indeed they had been given the impression that doing so was a luxury which, increasingly, they (and their colleagues) could not afford.

We cannot (and do not) claim these practical means are in any sense novel. We know people use them in reflective groups, peer review, learning sets, self-help groups, Balint-type groups and so on. So although these practical means were not original, in the context in which they were being used by our colleagues as a means for professional development and as a form of research, they were certainly novel.

We attempted, in providing the contributors with the means for freeing their practice, to give a lead. But in providing these practical means we did not intend them to be prescriptive. We fundamentally eschew a cook book approach to professional development. As Crissi said: "we can't give a prescription. All we can do is give an explanation of what we did. We've got to make clear the process we went through. We can only say what we felt was significant."

All we offered our colleagues was a set of tools to fashion something of their own making. Of course you might argue that the very nature of a tool determines what you can make with it. A paintbrush, a pen, and a chisel will produce quite different artefacts. So too theorising and autobiography will create quite different knowledge from a randomised controlled experiment. Our choice of tools was deliberate. Our belief was, and as a consequence of this project is even more strongly confirmed, that development of a professional's practice is much more likely to occur through their engaging in a process of insider practitioner research than through operating one form or another of traditional research. We are quite certain that the randomised control trial is unlikely to bring about much professional development whilst theorising one's practice and autobiographical writing almost certainly can. And these tools have created here, we believe, something quite unique – a collection that indicates the state of the health care professions today. Like other researchers the contributors have presented their data and we, like other research co-ordinators, have worked with those data to draw out some of their meanings as we have seen them. What the contributors have produced with the means we have offered them is now open to public scrutiny.

Secondly, at the theoretical level we believe we have contributed to the 'freeing up' of the contributors by exploring with them what we saw might be the theoretical and philosophical background to this kind of work. Not just this, but we have outlined much of this thinking in Chapters 3 and 4, where we explored Schön's distinction between the technical rational (TR) and professional artistry (PA) views of practice, and how TR views seriously constrain people's thinking, for example in areas such as the concept of expertise and theory, how to improve practice, and what is understood by quality. We drew on the work of Carr, developing Aristotle's distinction between theoretical and practical enquiry, and the difference Hoyle (and Stenhouse) make between extended and restricted professionals. We explored too the notion of case study research as a basis for insider practitioner research.

So, we provided the contributors with some theoretical frameworks for understanding the issues as they emerged. Thus, we discussed with them conventional approaches to research in health care (as described in Chapter 2), and a framework for clarifying our understanding of the nature of professional judgement (which we present in Chapter 13). We sensed that these frames of reference helped the contributors in the discussions we had with them, particularly once these discussions had taken place. As several of our contributors noted during the final workshop, if they had known much of the philosophical and theoretical basis of our approach before they had thought and written much, what they would have produced would have been very different and probably less worthwhile. It seems to us then that they might have arrived at too early a 'closure'. Whilst frames of reference which are offered to, rather than held by the practitioner, can help guide processes and make sense of issues once they have emerged, they are probably of limited value in providing a basis for gaining insight into one's *own* thinking and practice or of identifying those issues in the first place. But we recognise too (as did some – but not all – of our contributors) that formal theory has an important (even crucial) role to play in the development of practice, albeit after the practitioner has theorised his or her own personal practice. That is, it broadens and deepens the practitioner's insight. We noted that those of the contributors who made reference to formal theory in discussing their practice showed a deeper understanding of it than those who did not, and we suspect too that the effect of this on their future practice is likely to be greater.

But we have here something of a dilemma as editors of this book. Having said that formal theory is important and comes best after deliberation on practice, should we have included so much theory here, that is, before our *readers* have conducted much deliberation on *their* practice? Our defence would be twofold. Firstly we felt obliged to explain our theoretical basis to our colleagues during the project and that we should explain it to our readers. The difference of course is that some readers will have had the theory before engaging in very much practical discourse. Our concern is whether this will limit the scope of their own deliberations or restrict their insights. Our only comfort is that, if readers are much like our colleagues, reading the theory *before* the experience of deliberation will not make as much (or the same) sense as we hope it will by reading it *again* after engaging in some practical discourse. All we can hope, therefore, is that readers will return on some later occasion to what we have written, and reconsider it in the light of their own deliberations on practice.

The second justification we offer for including in this book some of the theoretical and philosophical basis of our work is that we felt constrained to lay out our stall as it were – to present our credentials. We acknowledge that some readers will have been sceptical about our approach, just as some of the contributors have. We recognise particularly that this might apply to people from a more conventional academic or research oriented background. We felt in writing this book rather like Becher and Kogan, who observed:

> The scientific paradigm has so successfully dominated social inquiry over the last half-century that any other approach is taken to demand an explanation, if not an apology. While we see no need for the second, we accept the obligation, in departing from strongly entrenched methodology, to put forward a more careful account of our rationale and our approach than would be expected of any staunchly positivistic and empirically based inquiry. (Becher and Kogan, 1980, p. 4)

So far we have looked at how this project freed up the contributors at a practical and a theoretical level. Now, thirdly, we should turn to its contribution at a personal level, which we found to be by far the most significant. But before examining this, perhaps we should look at the context of professional practice within which the contributors found themselves before the project began and which we described more fully in Chapters 1 and 2.

Like many of their own colleagues around them, our contributors were coping with a heavy service load and dealing with the inevitable stresses of a demanding, caring profession. They faced, too, the normal confusions and dilemmas of practice, and had to deal with the surprises that arise from time to time. Like other professionals they felt frustrated at not having the language or frameworks to articulate and validate their actions, let alone to explain or defend to others the reasons why they practised in the way they did. As we have already mentioned, two of our contributors even described themselves as feeling like frauds in this respect. Much of the foundation of their practice, they realised, was below the surface, hidden from view, and unrecognised even by themselves. As Clive put it "it's there, in our practice, but we've never been able to articulate it in the quick and easy way we can with the more public claims of professional practice. And we've never had the language. It's never been valued. Never been something we would sit down and talk about over coffee." Yet all the contributors recognised too that it was this hidden part of their practice that made them truly professionals, and was the very essence of their expertise.

In addition, the contributors felt overwhelmed by external pressures. Most saw themselves, initially at least, in conflict with what they came to construe as a technical rational view, endemic in much professional life anyway, and perhaps more so at the present time. They saw public and political forces demanding greater accountability of them and of other professions too. The trust once accorded by the public to professional people was no longer sufficient to sustain them, it seemed, and was being openly challenged. There was a culture now which demanded value for money, more for less, and perhaps worse, required health care to be 'delivered' through contracts with clearly defined outcome measures. Professionalism was becoming a technical matter, and they felt besieged by this because they intuitively felt it was untrue (but could not say why).

Though it did little to help their sense of frustration, the contributors saw some justice in certain of these claims. Much health care was, as they knew from their own experience, determined more by someone's whim or by tradition than by reasoned argument or evidence. A depressed patient, for example, might receive either electro-convulsive therapy or anti-depressant medication, perhaps remain in hospital five days rather than one, because the doctor said so or, more probably, because "we always do it this way". So when confronted by a more consumerist approach, many health professionals had colluded with public and politicians alike, partly because they knew there was waste and inefficiency in health care but more particularly because they were incapable of articulating what precisely they objected to regarding the newly emerging approach of 'contracted care'.

But there was a further reason why the contributors found this project helpful at a personal level. Beforehand very few of them had had much professional support provided either by their professional group or their employer. Certainly many professions are introducing continuing education schemes, and employers are beginning to introduce staff development schemes. In some professions there are reflective groups, clinical supervisors, mentoring schemes, preceptors for newly qualified staff, and some people form self-help groups or learning sets. But if our colleagues were at all typical of professionals at large, most of these initiatives had passed them by. As Richard said at the final workshop, "it's ironic that in all these years of practice this is the first time ever I've sat in a room with different professions and educationalists. I mean, it's unbelievable. Just having done that is a tremendous leap forward."

So, at the start of this project, the contributors presented themselves with what can only be described as low morale and reduced motivation, relatively high levels of stress, and unresolved tensions, confusions and dilemmas concerning their routine, day-to-day practice. It is also fair to say that they believed this was their inevitable 'lot' – the karma of the committed practitioner in the caring professions, at least for anyone who was not prepared to 'lower their sights' or to become cynical, or worse, to treat patients as inanimate objects, as diagnostic labels, as 'the broken leg in bed six'!

We must also report some of the contributors' reservations. Above all, the project took a long time. As Judith put it, "it's taken me a year to write one chapter", yet even then she saw this investment of time as necessary and perhaps reasonable in the context of her entire professional life. Others commented too that it was a process that needed time, and more especially time set aside specifically to engage in it. They felt too the weakness of their argument because, after all, what tangible results had they to show for their efforts? Discussion at this point quickly focused again on the contractual world they now worked in, and the insidious effects that outcome measures were having on their thinking. They felt, as Richard said, "sucked into the power game ... We are told every day we've got to produce outcomes, people are obsessed with outcomes, and this [project] doesn't fit with that."

Yet still the contributors felt their efforts would be realised in improved patient care. They were convinced that it must be – that it was being, and was paying off. Even feeling more committed to their professional practice was likely to be reflected in greater throughput, reduced wastage, and lower absenteeism. Clive put this well at the final workshop: "If you understand practice it must improve what you do. We have to start from the assumption that if we understand our practice it will improve what we do the rest of the time. If we don't value that as having some outcome ..."

They feared, too, that they might be seen as a special group, as different from others, people who were prepared to engage in such a project. They reflected that several of them had been sceptical at the start, and that all were very surprised at the worth of the project to them as individuals. Yet they also felt, from their experience with other colleagues, that people in the professions were also suspicious of present day consumerism and an overemphasis on outcome measures, speaking even of a 'ground swell of opinion', as one said, moving away from contracted care, of people wanting to find an alternative approach, sensing deep down that contracting would not improve care, that outcome measures were inappropriate for all areas of health, that there was a falseness about contracted care which did not feel right and did not accord with people's experience or beliefs in what professional people 'stood for'. Sheila summed this up for the others at the final workshop: "We are not unusual. I don't think I am unusual. Oh, I knew about it [reflective practice] but I was very sceptical about it. And I didn't have time for it. Oh, I know the reasons why that was, but the more it comes out in the open the more you realise everyone wants to be able to talk and comment about these issues, rather than things about outcomes. It's just we've never learnt how to do it. We've never been told it was important to do it. So we don't do it."

The contributors recognised too that others might be more difficult to convince about the value of this approach, and indeed that some might never be convinced. And they also recognised that you cannot convince others simply by describing your experience to them or by telling them of its value for you. People have to experience this for themselves. They felt the right conditions must be created for people to find value in the process. There is a need for a supportive environment. So the contributors recognised an eternal dilemma: you need a supportive culture for this process to be effective, yet engaging in the process can make a significant contribution to developing the very same supportive culture.

So what then was the contribution of this project at a personal level to the contributors? Repeatedly we have used the term 'freed', and we have done so deliberately. The contributors' overwhelming view, we sensed, was that by going through this process, they felt liberated, unconstrained, released in some strange way from what can only be described as some kind of 'bondage' in their professional lives up to then. Not just this, but they felt the process had legitimised aspects of their professional work which until then they had felt diffident about articulating or explaining to others. More than this, up to now they simply did not have the language to do so. The hidden element of their practice that they so often referred to was now very real for them. It had been revealed. They could see it, it was palpable, and they saw its basis, its foundation, its fundamentals. They now saw that it was quite legitimate to spend time and effort on a process of reflection and deliberation on their practice. It had to be. The project had shown it was acceptable *and* worthwhile.

But if the contributors sensed they had been freed, they also felt more confident. They had been prepared at the outset to attempt this deliberation on their practice. They had stuck to their task, even with its ups and downs, blind alleys, and false starts. They kept re-visiting areas of their work (and of themselves) they had never expected to visit. And they had gone further and further into it. As Sheila said, "for me it was looking at an aspect of my practice which I would never have bothered to look at before. It was too messy, too nasty. I would have said to myself: 'I don't want to talk about that, you've got to get on. Who cares about that? That's happened, it's over and done with, you've got to get on, get on with the next thing.' But for me, looking at it, it became an exciting experience, eventually – once I'd got through the difficulty of facing up to it. Usually we don't articulate it, and it's because no-one has shown us how to do it. But more particularly no-one has told us it's worth doing. Not just that it's OK to do it but, hey, why haven't we done it before?"

Importantly the group gained significant insights into their practice and perhaps especially into themselves. Above all the project was enlightening, it shed light for them, it was illuminating, and this was enlivening; people felt energised, more motivated. They began to see the world of their practice differently. They had developed new frameworks for seeing things. And they saw themselves differently too but they were not 'empowered' by their experiences. They had not become, in Grundy's (1987) term, 'emancipated'. They felt there was too much power in health care already, and they did not want to be "sucked into the power game". Nor did they want to fight politics with politics. There had to be another way, a quite different way, and they felt they had found it in the enlightenment they had achieved.

Certainly they saw professionalism differently by the end of the project. They saw themselves truly as professional people. They understood their own personal basis of the profession in which they had spent their working life. They saw a oneness of themselves, their practice and their profession. They saw themselves more as individuals, within the traditions of their practice. They were more in control of themselves, and of their practice, of their professionalism.

Expertise took on a new meaning too. They began to recognise that true expertise lay in that part of their practice which until then had been hidden from view. Clive introduced the metaphor of the iceberg in Chapter 10. Being expert now meant recognising this fact, and devoting time and effort to exposing and exploring that hidden realm of one's professional practice. Being an expert meant understanding as fully as possible the basis of one's practice, yet paradoxically recognising that you never fully can, that there will always be more to reveal, further insights to be gained. Being expert (as opposed to being *an* expert) – that is having some expertise – meant undertaking a continual exploration. As Clive put it at the final workshop, "it's validating this way of working, and understanding the complexities of our practice. Lifelong learning is either a cliché (which it probably is) or it's a commitment to go on with it, with its ups and downs."

The iceberg metaphor for professional practice is worth taking a little further (see Figure 14.1). The part of it 'above the surface' which we actually see comprises our professional 'doing' and 'saying'. It is the activities of professional daily life – our busy-ness. And frequently, as our colleagues reminded us, we are so busy with all this that we often do not stop to question it. On or about the water level of the professional iceberg is our experiencing of our practice, our awareness that we are doing and saying things in certain ways, often without thinking. Some of this experiencing we are aware of (and is above the surface). Some we are not (and is below). We might have the experience but miss the meaning. Just below the surface lies our knowledge – our personal knowledge or 'know-how', made up of personal theory, influenced of course by formal theory yet distinct from it too. And further down are our assumptions and expectations, all bedded onto our beliefs and values.

The significance of the iceberg metaphor goes even further. As we 'do' more and more we risk top loading our iceberg, and make it unstable so that it is likely to capsize. It is the area 'below the surface' that gives our practice stability and buoyancy, and we need to spend time building up our hidden expertise if we wish to improve. Yet this aspect of our practice is hidden from view, below the surface, hidden not just from others (who only see the doing and saying) but it is most likely to be hidden from ourselves too. The true expert, then, is someone who knows something of what

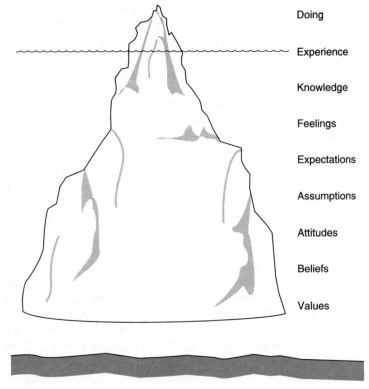

Figure 14.1   The iceberg of professional practice

lies beneath the surface of his or her practice, and spends time and effort not just understanding it but developing it further, and who can then talk about it more publicly too. In all these senses he or she is the extended professional we speak of in Chapter 4.

In short, the contributors felt that this project had changed them as people. They were seeing themselves anew. They were under-standing and discovering new things about their own practice. They felt that as a result they would be better prepared for the unexpected. They did not feel that necessarily they would know precisely how they would practise differently, even if situations like the ones they described in their incidents were repeated. They did not have an 'action plan'; they had not worked out what they would do differently or how they would improve. They would not have *the* answer, or know what was *right*. They recognised that perhaps there would never be 'the answer' or 'the right thing' to do. But they were sure that they knew how to explore a range of options, and felt more confident in making professional judgements in 'weighing up' the situation. There would always be tensions between perhaps equally valid alternatives, where they were the only person in the situation who could make the decision. But they felt more confident they would do this, and be better at living with the consequences.

They recognised that there would be further conflicts and tensions, more confusions, further stresses for them in their professional life. This was inevitable. But they now saw that these were normal. They now knew these confusions did not occur because they were not being professional enough. They were not a sign of weakness on their part. It was not that they had been inadequately educated. It was not that, given time, they would 'get there in the end'.

But they did recognise that these confusions and tensions could be resolved; that they could be reflected upon; that there had to be deliberation on their practice; that time and effort had to be devoted to this; that these deliberations should be on everyone's agenda – theirs, their colleagues', their managers', that of the commissioners of health care, and on the agenda of patients and clients. But, above all, resolving these confusions and tensions was something which only they could do for themselves. This project had given them back their professionalism.

References

Becher, T. and Kogan, M. (1980). *Process and Structure in Higher Education*. Heinemann Educational.

Grundy, S. (1987). *Curriculum: Product or Praxis?* Falmer Press.

Schön, D. A. (1983). *The Reflective Practitioner*. Basic Books.

Chapter 15

Insider practitioner research: a way ahead

Introduction

In the previous chapter we discussed the process which led the contributors to write about their practice, and we listed the outcomes for them and for us as editors of this book. Now we turn to the wider implications of this work.

Our conclusions can be simply stated: professional practice truly develops when practitioners research their own practice. But what does this mean? Why do we say this, and how can it come about? These are the questions we will address in this final chapter.

In Part One of this book we described the state of the health care professions at the end of the twentieth century. Professional people, we said, are under siege – they are caught between powerful opposing forces. On the one hand they see a world demanding greater value for money and accountability, where their autonomy is threatened, and their professional actions are being brought under control. On the other hand, they know intuitively that professional people need autonomy; that professionalism is hugely complex; that being a professional is so much more than the acquisition of certain skills or a set of competencies. Yet they are aware too that they cannot easily explain the need for this autonomy, why they require such a lengthy education, and why they should be trusted.

What this project demonstrated to the contributors was this.

- They felt unprepared by their education to cope with the

unexpected and unplanned-for aspects of their practice, yet they recognised this to be the very essence of professionalism.

- They were surprised to realise the complex nature of their practice, and to recognise that their expertise was largely intuitive – hidden not just from others but from themselves.
- They discovered that their practice was as much based on their personal knowledge as it was on formal (outside) knowledge, and that being presented with new (outside) knowledge often failed to change their (and their colleagues') practice.
- They came to see that their practice developed when they understood more clearly their personal knowledge, and saw how powerfully this acts as a barrier to the adopting of new ideas.
- As a consequence, they felt more confident in their practice, more able to give an account of it and defend it, more reassured of the basis of their professional actions, and more able (and prepared) to change their practice because they had questioned (and where necessary modified) their personal knowledge.

So this project demonstrated to the contributors (and confirmed for us) that the struggle professionals were facing was not between opposing forces; that the problem in fact lay elsewhere; that the question that needs to be addressed is not how can professionals maintain their autonomy in the face of increasing bureaucratic control, but rather how can professionals be held accountable for their practice if they are unable satisfactorily to give an account of it?

Insider practitioner research

The contribution of this project, then, has been to introduce to the contributors what we have termed insider practitioner research – professionals researching their own practice. To be sure it is an ungainly term but we can find no satisfactory alternative at the present time. Table 15.1 shows its major features (and can usefully be compared to the four research traditions we explored in Chapter 2, Table 2.1, p. 23).

Examples of insider practitioner research include critical incident analysis, video recordings of one's practice, and case studies. Its scope is the individual practitioner's world, and its purposes are to

Table 15.1   Insider practitioner research: a new research tradition for the professions

	Insider practitioner research
Examples	Critical incident analysis, video of practice, case study
Scope	The individual practitioner's world
Purposes	To understand the knowledge, personal theory, beliefs, assumptions, expectations, and values that underpin one's own practice, and through this to improve it
Scale	Self
Interest served	Practitioner (and hence practice) development
Development metaphor	Enlightenment

understand the knowledge and personal theory that underpin one's practice, and through this to improve it. Insider practitioner research is conducted by practitioners on themselves, and primarily serves the interest of the practitioner in developing his or her practice. As a metaphor for development which arises from insider practitioner research we have chosen the term 'enlightenment'. This we believe was the outcome for our colleagues, and we would argue is the most significant outcome for practitioners of any research since it is only through personal enlightenment that professionals' practice improves.

Insider practitioner research does not require the researcher (that is, the practitioner) to be an expert in research itself. Rather, it requires the practitioner (who *is* in fact the researcher) to bring to the research his or her own practical expertise, for this is the very focus of the research process. Indeed, all health care professionals at any stage of their development (including – crucially – during the undergraduate phase of their education) can engage in it. Practitioners are simply asked to bring to it some aspect of their practice (for example, an experience of their practice). The research process then proceeds as we described in the previous chapters.

We are certain, too, that insider practitioner research is valuable in any aspect of professional practice, from apparently simple skills (such as suture tying in surgery), through apparently technical procedures (such as washing a patient), to the more obviously complex interpersonal actions (such as breaking bad news). In all of these examples, practice is underpinned with personal theory, large elements of which are often hidden but which can be unearthed and critically appreciated.

How can this come about?

The major constraint to insider practitioner research is time. However, we believe this is less of a challenge than it seems. We would not demand *more* time for this but the redeployment of existing time.

During the undergraduate phase of education, many health care students are expected to conduct a project of one sort or another. Typically these adopt one form or another of the traditional research approaches we described in Chapter 2. They could (and we argue should) involve insider practitioner research, with students looking into aspects of practice they are experiencing. Qualified practitioners are expected to undertake audit, and some more formally engage in research. Again, the time could be used for insider practitioner research which would itself contribute to audit (and could even be claimed truly to be audit). Continuing professional development often means attending conferences, lectures and seminars, which are of questionable benefit to the development of practice (Davis *et al.*, 1995). Much of this time could more usefully be spent on insider practitioner research. And the time currently spent (by some) on the preparation of clinical guidelines and protocols could similarly be used (we believe more profitably) by all practitioners. Indeed, the evidence suggests that by doing this practitioners' practice is more likely to develop than by being issued guidelines and protocols (Davis *et al.*, 1995).

In addition to finding the time, this work must be valued by key people within the organisation. They are professionals too, and their professional expertise also lies beneath the surface. By conducting insider practitioner research *themselves*, they will come to recognise its value to them and to others. In this way, an 'evaluative culture' (Haines and Jones, 1994) will be created in which professionals are constantly looking at what they do and learning from this.

But if these are some of the practical aspects of implementing insider practitioner research, how can it be introduced? We believe there is an important role here for outsiders. But not for outsiders who remain outside, rather outsiders who become insiders.

Traditionally this 'outside' role has been an academic function – to conduct research, to discover new knowledge, to promulgate the findings, and for practitioners to apply these to their practice. But this approach has failed to influence practice (Haines and Jones, 1994). Hence our insistence that insider practitioner research is necessary. As Stenhouse said in relation to the development of teaching in schools: academics have a contribution to make; 'but it is the teachers who in the end will change the world of the school by understanding it' (Stenhouse, 1975, p. 208). His vision was of schools 'as research and development institutions rather than clients of research and development agencies' (p. 223). He saw the role of academics 'as helping schools to undertake research and development in a problem area and to report this work in a way that supports similar developments in other schools' (p. 223). He added 'a research tradition which is accessible to teachers and which feeds teaching must be created if education is to be significantly improved' (p. 165).

We believe the same is true for the professions involved in health care. A similar tradition needs to be established, and this can occur through insider practitioner research. This will require a close partnership between academics and professional practitioners, a partnership of equals. But this requires a new approach by academics. Eraut sums this up when he suggests that the barriers to linking the academic world and the world of practice 'are most likely to be overcome if higher education is prepared to extend its role from that of creator and transmitter of generalisable knowledge to that of *enhancing the knowledge-creating capacities* of individuals and professional communities' (Eraut, 1994, p. 57).

The contributors recognised that through this project (by understanding their practice and the hidden expertise which underpins it) they were conducting insider practitioner research. But more than this, they were developing their practice, and engaging in education at *one and the same time*. More particularly, they recognised that they were researching, educating and developing themselves. A synthesis of education, research and practice development had occurred. And they recognised too, that if all practitioners were to undertake insider practitioner research, at all levels, and throughout their careers from first year undergraduate to the day of their retirement, then – in a very real sense – professional education would be occurring.

So our conclusion from this project which has engaged six of our colleagues from different health professions in thinking and writing about their practice is that professional education and practice development are one and the same. They are united by insider practitioner research. This integration, in theory and in practice, occurs when professionals undertake work such as we have described in this book, that is, when they expose and explore, make explicit and articulate, the hidden basis of their professional practice. This requires a dynamic partnership, yet a partnership of equals, between academics (outsiders) and practitioners (insiders). Through this partnership practitioners will develop a clearer understanding of themselves and their practice, and through this, the practice in which they engage will become enhanced.

References

Davis, D. A., Thomson, M. A., Oxman, A. D. and Haynes, R. B. (1995). Changing physician performance, a systematic review of the effect of continuing medical education strategies. *Journal of the American Medical Association*, **274**, 700–705.

Eraut, M. (1994). *Developing Professional Knowledge and Competence*. Falmer Press.

Haines, A. and Jones, R. (1994). Implementing findings of research. *British Medical Journal*, **308**, 1488–1492.

Stenhouse, L. (1975). *An Introduction to Curriculum Research and Development*. Heinemann.

Index